Nursing History
for Contemporary
Role Development

Sandra B. Lewenson, EdD, RN, FAAN, coeditor of the book, *Capturing Nursing History: A Guide to Historical Methods in Nursing,* is a professor of nursing at Pace University, College of Health Professions in Pleasantville, New York. She teaches in the master of nursing education program as well as the graduate core courses where she integrates history into the courses she teaches. She has developed both a master's and an undergraduate course in nursing history that has evolved into an online course. Dr. Lewenson has published widely on nursing's political activity during the first half of the 20th century and on the history of public health nursing and primary health care. She is the recipient of the American Association for the History of Nursing (AAHN) 1995 Lavinia Dock Award for Exemplary Research and Writing for her book, *Taking Charge: Nursing Suffrage and Feminism, 1873–1920,* and received the Mary M. Roberts Award for Exemplary Writing (2013) for her edited book (coedited with Patricia D'Antonio) *Nursing Interventions Through Time: History as Evidence.* Dr. Lewenson has coedited *Public Health Nursing: Practicing Population-Based Care,* as well as the most recently published *Practicing Primary Health Care in Nursing: Caring for Populations,* with Marie Truglio-Londrigan. In 2016, the Nursing Education Alumni Association at Teachers College, Columbia University, awarded her the prestigious R. Louise McManus Medal for her leadership in nursing.

Annemarie McAllister, EdD, RN, dean of the Cochran School of Nursing at St. John's Riverside in Yonkers, New York, has taught an online nursing history course to undergraduate students and graduate core courses with historical components at Pace University, College of Health Professions in Pleasantville, New York. Her research focuses on the history of the associate degree program as it was designed at Teachers College, Columbia University, in New York City during the mid-20th century. Her work explores the development of curricula at the associate degree level and the success of the leaders who were the proponents of this educational program, including Mildred Montag and R. Louise McManus. She received the American Association for the History of Nursing (AAHN) H31 Pre-Doctoral Research Grant Award to complete her dissertation titled, *R. Louise McManus and Mildred Montag Create the Associate Degree Model for the Education of Nurses: The Right Leaders, the Right Time, the Right Place: 1947–1959.* In 2013, she was awarded the prestigious AAHN Teresa Christy Award for Exemplary Research and Writing for her outstanding contribution to nursing. She recently published two chapters, "Inside Track of Doing Historical Research: My Dissertation Story" and "Learning the Historical Method: Step by Step," in *Nursing Research Using Historical Methods: Qualitative Designs and Methods in Nursing,* edited by Mary de Chesnay (Springer Publishing).

Kylie M. Smith, PhD, joined the Nell Hodgson Woodruff School of Nursing at Emory University as the school's first Andrew W. Mellon Faculty Fellow in Nursing and the Humanities, in November 2015. Dr. Smith's research focuses on American psychiatric nursing history, particularly approaches to advanced practice in the context of the Cold War. Prior to joining Emory, she served as lecturer at the School of Nursing at the University of Wollongong, Australia, where she taught reflective practice and incorporated humanities research and teaching methods into nursing curricula. In 2014, Dr. Smith received the prestigious Karen Buhler Wilkerson fellowship from the Barbara Bates Center for the Study of the History of Nursing at the University of Pennsylvania to undertake research into the development of American psychiatric nursing after World War II. This research has been further supported by grants from the Rockefeller Archive Center in New York and the American Association for the History of Nursing (AAHN). In 2015, she received the AAHN H15 Award for her current research, which looks at the relationships among American psychiatry, nurses, and race in the mid-20th century.

Nursing History
for Contemporary
Role Development

SANDRA B. LEWENSON, EdD, RN, FAAN
ANNEMARIE MCALLISTER, EdD, RN
KYLIE M. SMITH, PhD

Editors

SPRINGER PUBLISHING COMPANY
NEW YORK

Springer Publishing Company, LLC
11 West 42nd Street
New York, NY 10036
www.springerpub.com

Acquisitions Editor: Joseph Morita
Production Editor: Kris Parrish
Composition: Westchester Publishing Services

ISBN: 978-0-8261-3237-6
e-book ISBN: 978-0-8261-3238-3
Instructor's Manual ISBN: 978-0-8261-3239-0

Instructor's Materials are available to qualified adopters by contacting textbook@springerpub.com

16 17 18 19 20 / 5 4 3 2 1

The author and the publisher of this Work have made every effort to use sources believed to be reliable to provide information that is accurate and compatible with the standards generally accepted at the time of publication. Because medical science is continually advancing, our knowledge base continues to expand. Therefore, as new information becomes available, changes in procedures become necessary. We recommend that the reader always consult current research and specific institutional policies before performing any clinical procedure. The author and publisher shall not be liable for any special, consequential, or exemplary damages resulting, in whole or in part, from the readers' use of, or reliance on, the information contained in this book. The publisher has no responsibility for the persistence or accuracy of URLs for external or third-party Internet websites referred to in this publication and does not guarantee that any content on such websites is, or will remain, accurate or appropriate.

Library of Congress Cataloging-in-Publication Data

Names: Lewenson, Sandra B., editor. | McAllister, Annemarie, 1957– editor. | Smith, Kylie M., editor.
Title: Nursing history for contemporary role development / Sandra B. Lewenson, Annemarie McAllister, Kylie M. Smith, editors.
Description: New York, NY : Springer Publishing Company, LLC, [2017] | Includes bibliographical references.
Identifiers: LCCN 2016036306 (print) | LCCN 2016037359 (ebook) | ISBN 9780826132376 (hardcopy : alk. paper) | ISBN 9780826132383 (eBook) | ISBN 9780826132390 (Instructor's manual) | ISBN 9780826132383 (ebook)
Subjects: | MESH: History of Nursing | Nurse's Role—history | Ethics, Nursing—history | History, 20th Century | United States
Classification: LCC RT42 (print) | LCC RT42 (ebook) | NLM WY 11 AA1 | DDC 610.73—dc23
LC record available at https://lccn.loc.gov/2016036306

Printed in the United States of America by Gasch Printing.

Contents

Contributors

Susan Benedict, DSN, CRNA, FAAN
Assistant Dean
The University of Texas Health Science Center at Houston
School of Nursing
Houston, Texas

Geertje Boschma, PhD, RN
Professor
University of British Columbia, School of Nursing
Vancouver, British Columbia, Canada

Jane Brooks, PhD, RN
Senior Lecturer
Unit Lead for Core Values for Professional Nursing
Master of Research Examinations' Officer
University of Manchester School of Nursing
Manchester, England

J. Margo Brooks Carthon, PhD, APRN, FAAN
Assistant Professor of Nursing
University of Pennsylvania School of Nursing
Philadelphia, Pennsylvania

Karen Flynn, PhD
Associate Professor of Gender and Women's Studies
Associate Professor for African American Studies
University of Illinois at Urbana-Champaign
Urbana, Illinois

Mary Eckenrode Gibson, PhD, RN
Associate Professor of Nursing
Assistant Director, Bjoring Center for Nursing Historical Inquiry
University of Virginia School of Nursing
Charlottesville, Virginia

Sandra B. Lewenson, EdD, RN, FAAN
Professor
Pace University College of Health Professions
Lienhard School of Nursing
Pleasantville, New York

Linda Tina Maldonado, PhD, RN
Assistant Professor
Villanova University College of Nursing
Villanova, Pennsylvania

April D. Matthias, PhD, RN, CNE
Assistant Professor
University of North Carolina Wilmington School of Nursing
Wilmington, North Carolina

Annemarie McAllister, EdD, RN
Dean
Cochran School of Nursing
Yonkers, New York

Linda Shields, MD (Research), PhD, RN, FACN, FAAN,
  Centaur Fellow MAICD
Professor of Nursing
School of Nursing Midwifery and Indigenous Health
Charles Sturt University, Bathurst, New South Wales
Honorary Professor, School of Medicine
The University of Queensland
Brisbane, Queensland, Australia

Briana Ralston Smith, PhD, RN
Fellow, Barbara Bates Center for the Study of the History of Nursing
University of Pennsylvania School of Nursing
Philadelphia, Pennsylvania

Kylie M. Smith, PhD
Assistant Professor
Andrew W. Mellon Faculty Fellow for Nursing and the Humanities
Nell Hodgson Woodruff School of Nursing
Senior Faculty Fellow
Emory Center for Ethics
Emory University
Atlanta, Georgia

Barbra Mann Wall, PhD, RN, FAAN
Thomas A. Saunders III Professorship in Nursing
University of Virginia School of Nursing
Charlottesville, Virginia

Foreword

Joan Lynaugh, my mentor and dear friend, said, "everything has a past." As this book, *Nursing History for Contemporary Role Development*, edited by Sandra B. Lewenson, Annemarie McAllister, and Kylie M. Smith, wisely shows, the nursing profession indeed has an important past. Nurses have been a part of every social movement, conflict zone, institutional change, and aspect of care from the moment of individuals' illnesses to their attempts and successes protecting their health, to their deaths. That past is a critical part of our ability to understand how our current roles as nursing professionals changed over time, and how we might think about them in the future. Our past shapes everything we do, whether we explicitly acknowledge it or not.

It is important to remember our past. We sometimes think our modern roles are extraordinary and new, that what we do as clinicians, educators, and policy decision makers has no bearing on or does not draw from the past. We would be misguided to think this way and to forget that although the context has changed, our clinical and policy decisions are fundamentally steeped in the past. For example, as we focus our practices, educational programs, and policy on the culture of health, we would be remiss to forget that nurses throughout their history have tried to mediate the effects of poverty on health, as well as educate patients about the health benefits of clean air and good nutrition. School nurses, mental health nurses, and public health and rural nurses in particular understood the importance of the environment and the family to the health of an individual (although there are also examples of nurses who were biased, racist, and classist). Today, the context and the language are different. We have sometimes forgotten and minimized our focus on the social determinants of health—for example, our educational programs and practice since the 1950s rested on acute care—but these factors, in the context of our fragmented and expensive health system, are becoming more prominent in our health policies today. We have a renewed recognition of how social determinants of health do inform how we treat and engage patients over a continuum of care, as several of the chapters in this book illustrate.

Technology is another example of how our past practices inform our present and future. I recently attended a symposium on innovation in nursing. All were excited to see what they could develop from a kit of circuit boards, bands, and other pieces of equipment, but few knew the history of nurses' innovations. By understanding our history, we know that nurses inventing new devices and models of care, or repurposing typical materials and devices to better care for their patients, is not new, but a constant factor in the way nurses protected their patients and improved their patients' care. Nurses, as we see in this volume, created new models of care, developed "work arounds" to make equipment work better, and reorganized care to protect their most vulnerable patients. Perhaps because nursing has traditionally been characterized as a woman's profession under medical control, new ideas and making things work have not typically been recognized as "nursing innovation." Our practice and our educational programs covertly and overtly teach students about the opportunities of creativity and idea generation, but without the historical context, each device or model seems new and untethered to larger social and cultural structures and meanings.

As we think about how our professional and disciplinary roles will change over the next decades, it would be wise to remember that how we practice, educate, and influence policy today will inform the future. Today's work is tomorrow's history. Our profession and our patients are critically dependent upon future nurses, how they are educated, and how and where they practice. Our history must be a key part of any curriculum we offer, and provide the foundation for new ideas and instill meaning for our practice and policy making. Indeed, "everything has a past," but we need to know our history, embrace it, and build on it. This is exactly the purpose and the mission of this book. It provides students with a foundation to know about the past, understand the present, and think about the future. This book also provides a rich resource and opportunity for faculty who might not be well versed in their profession's history to integrate history into their courses across all content areas and program levels. It provides a "lifeline" from the past to the future, nicely illustrating why an understanding of the past situates us to better shape our future.

Julie Fairman, PhD, RN, FAAN
Chair, Biobehavioral Health Sciences Department
Nightingale Professor of Nursing
Director Emerita, Barbara Bates Center for the Study
of the History of Nursing
Co-Director, Robert Wood Johnson Foundation Future
of Nursing Scholars Program
University of Pennsylvania School of Nursing
Philadelphia, Pennsylvania

"We older nurses look to you to do better than we have done," said Lillian Wald, the noted leader of public health nursing, in an address she gave to the 1918 graduating class of the Johns Hopkins School of Nursing (Wald, 1918a, p. 12). She turned to these new nurses in hopes of a better future. Women in America still did not yet have the vote, and World War I was slowly abating, leaving a trail of social disruption. Access to better health care for those in urban and rural settings, along with political equality, Wald believed, needed to be something for nurses to work toward. That same year, Wald (1918b) wrote, "women should support with their political influence the taxation and legislation which are needed for the establishment and the maintenance of visiting and public health nurses since the health of the community rests largely with such nurses" (p. 1). She, like other nursing pioneers, linked nursing and politics with better health care outcomes. Her political beliefs, along with her nursing knowledge and her ability to inform the public, provide lessons for nurses today who seek similar goals of health care for all. Wald looked to the new graduates to lead the way toward a better future where there would be public and private support for new nursing initiatives. These students took courses in nursing history where they learned of the early nurse leaders, such as Wald herself, and the obstacles these pioneers overcame. The link between nursing and political advocacy was made explicit to students, as it was considered central to improving the health of the public and achieving the future that Wald envisioned.

The question, then, for students of today is how do we make that link between nursing and political advocacy for the patients, families, communities, and populations in our care? How do we find our place among the many roles that nurses undertake today in the practice, education, and research arenas? One response to these questions can be to look at our history. History informs us of who we are, where we came from, what we are doing now, and even where we are going. But there is more to nursing history than this. Nursing history matters because of nursing's history, because it is that history that has so sharply defined and shaped and even constrained the profession we know today. We need to know the mistakes that have been made so we can try not to make them again. We need to know the victories, to remind ourselves of what this profession is capable. Yet if we were to ask most nurses today what they know about nursing history, they are hard pressed to name anyone of note beyond Florence Nightingale. Nightingale's impact on nursing cannot be denied, but her "heroic" legacy threatens to overshadow the reality of the profession she helped to create, and the multitude of women (for they were mostly women) who made the ancient work of caring for the sick into the complex set of practices that it is today. In their article "History Counts," Julie Fairman and Patricia D'Antonio set out explicitly the ways in which today's health care systems, policies, and practices, which are often regarded as timeless and inevitable, are in fact shaped by both deliberate choices and exigent circumstances over which nurses sometimes had no control, and over which they sometimes did (Fairman & D'Antonio, 2013). Understanding the historical forces that have shaped contemporary nursing facilitates a critical analysis of the assumptions, often taken for granted, that underpin contemporary health systems. Within these systems, nurses have been self-consciously active in the making of their own profession, the work they do, and the circumstances under which they do it; and we are not at the end of that process.

WHY WRITE THIS BOOK?

Nursing history scholarship is a rapidly growing field with new and exciting work emerging about nursing's past and its impact on the present. For students and faculty dealing with already laden curricula, often focused on techno-rational clinical competencies, engaging with historical scholarship can be seen as overwhelming and difficult. A number of nursing scholars from around the world have previously demonstrated that finding ways to bring historical elements into nursing curricula is needed, and that the benefits to students are manifold (D'Antonio, Connolly, Wall, Whelan, & Fairman, 2010; Lewenson, 2004;

McAllister, John, & Gray, 2009; McAllister, Madsen, Godden, Greenhill, & Reed, 2010; Smith, Brown, & Crookes, 2015; Toman & Thifault, 2012). This book aims to address this need in an accessible and innovative way, summarizing existing histories and showcasing the work of emerging nursing history scholars that may not be available elsewhere. In this way, we hope to stimulate the interest and intellect of students in nursing to help them understand the relevance of historical context for all aspects of nursing and health care. The book helps faculty and students access and apply historical research to current issues in nursing education, research, and practice, as well as reflect on the enduring themes currently found in nursing and health care. And as students develop an understanding of what history can offer them, they, too, may become interested in becoming historians of the future.

WHAT IS UNIQUE ABOUT THIS BOOK?

Nursing History for Contemporary Role Development identifies a number of significant issues relevant to the complexities of contemporary nursing, and examines the background of those issues within the context of time and place. It then relates these historical findings to contemporary practice, drawing on the scholarship of expert historians to unravel the ways in which that practice has developed. In this way, the book provides a unique depth and breadth to our understanding of approaches to human health that are relevant for nurses and other health professionals as they work toward a healthier society.

The chapters in the book address key themes in contemporary nursing practice, providing evidence of how nursing fits within the broader context of culture and society, from the late 19th century to the present. The book uses historical case studies that relate to specific issues in the development of the profession. The contributing authors introduce their chapters with a contemporary issue, and then provide the contextual background for the reader to understand. The case studies provide a springboard for each chapter's further discussion and conclusion. The chapters address issues, such as how certain specializations in the profession evolved, how nurses have been educated, how differentiation of practice affects health outcomes, how nurses have engaged in health care policy and political advocacy addressing vulnerable populations, how legal and ethical issues affected practice, and how nurses provided care during wartime. The rights of vulnerable populations, whether in the community or in schools, in the newly formed neonatal intensive care units (NICUs), in mental institutions, in academia, or in war zones, resonate throughout this work and raise questions about nursing roles during contemporary times.

This book provides students with the historical context that otherwise may not be readily available to them, making explicit this connection between the past and the present. By drawing on the expert scholarship of historians, and using primary source case studies, it also provides a rich tool with which to facilitate self-reflection, socialization, and decision-making skills essential for students and all nurses. The chapters in this book include questions at the end requiring reflective and critical thinking, making history readily accessible to students in their education and, therefore, their subsequent practice.

The editors conceived of this book to be used by all students of nursing and all nurses. *Nursing History for Contemporary Role Development* supports students in undergraduate and accelerated programs and enriches students in master's and doctoral programs. In academia, educators designing curricula for undergraduate, graduate, and doctoral programs will find this book a useful resource. Undergraduate students need an understanding of nursing and health care history so they can appreciate how nursing fits into society, how the profession evolved within the context of societal norms and issues, and what it means for their own development as leaders within the profession. The chapters in this book help graduate and prelicensure students explore the development of the advanced practice role, licensure and registration issues, and how nursing relates to social and health care legislation over time (e.g., Medicaid, Medicare, the Affordable Care Act, and other historical and contemporary social reform acts). Students engaged in doctoral research can use this book to facilitate analysis of the ethical, political, and leadership issues that shape their future practice; for example, considering the long-term ramifications of nurses participating in government-sanctioned ethnic cleansing, or understanding why there are three educational pathways into nursing practice and what this means for the future. These issues and more are addressed in this text and allow students at all levels to read about an issue, consider what has been published in the literature, explore a related historical exemplar, and then consider the implications of this history for the future.

And finally, we see the audience as those nurses in clinical settings where a historical framework can provide depth and breadth to past practice, current issues, and futuristic thinking. Critical thinking and clinical reasoning "at the bedside" can be informed by a historical sensibility that seeks to question routines and procedures that are sometimes taken for granted, negotiate ethical and interpersonal issues in health care systems, and understand patients in the context of their whole lives, as a product of their society.

ORGANIZATION OF THE BOOK

Nursing History for Contemporary Role Development invited expert historians of nursing from around the world to contribute a chapter. These authors write about a key theme in contemporary practice and include historical case studies to be used for knowledge translation. The 11 chapters are organized into four sections, according to the time of the historical story. Earlier historical context is given in the various sections, creating a rich tapestry that spans time and space.

In Section I, the authors explore issues concerning diversity, vulnerable populations, and the rise of nursing specialties. Themes addressed in this section include being part of a minority population and what that means to health care or lack of health care. Another theme explores the origins of public health nursing, specifically examining rural public health nursing and the American Red Cross. The third theme in this section expands on the role of school nurses in rural America. Overlapping historical background adds richness to these first three chapters in the book and provides a foundation of what happens in later years.

In Chapter 1, J. Margo Brooks Carthon addresses the health care needs of the African American community in Philadelphia, a community that faced lack of adequate housing, racism, and poor access to care. Similar to today, minority communities continued to experience the untoward effect of insufficient access to health care laced with pervasive racial bias and a lack of a diverse workforce, all of which adversely affected the quality and safety of the health care offered and the health care outcomes obtained. Carthon uses the historical exemplar of Mary Elizabeth Tyler, a minority public health nurse, at the turn of the 20th century in Philadelphia to describe how diversity in nursing positively affected the health care outcomes of a community. The Whittier Centre, a philanthropic association in Philadelphia, addressed the Black community's efforts to combat a tuberculosis outbreak in the city. This organization hired a Black nurse to work and live within the community to serve as a liaison between the community and the Whittier Centre. The success of her work during that period provides, first, an historical account of public health nursing, specifically, the contributions of minority nurses in this area. Second, it offers contemporary nurses an opportunity to be reflective about the need for a diverse workforce that will care for an increasingly diverse population. It forces us to consider the possibilities of what has happened in the past and the ways in which a diverse workforce can improve the health care for all today.

When we see reports concerning public health issues in current media sources, they are often presented as if they are new and in need of new public health strategies. In Chapter 2, Sandra B. Lewenson examines the long-held role of the public health nurse through the lens of the larger framework of primary health care. Using Healthy People 2020 (2016) that laid out goals for a healthier nation, Lewenson argues that public health nurses should work together with community activists in order to provide the resources needed to meet the health needs of the community.

Lewenson presents an early 20th-century effort to address the health needs of a small rural community in upstate New York. The leadership in the town of Red Hook joined forces with the American Red Cross in the early 20th century and determined the needs of the community using data collected in a door-to-door survey of the town. Using these data, the town partnered with the American Red Cross's rural public health service called Town and Country Nursing Service and created strategies to provide for the health and well-being of this rural population. This case study demonstrates how community leaders worked together with public health nurses using evidence-based data as a basis for planning for the needs of the community. As contemporary public health nurses work within a broad primary health care framework to achieve the goals outlined in Healthy People 2020, their roles include collaboration with many participants both locally and nationally. The efforts of the leaders of a small, rural town in upstate New York in the early 20th century to provide for the health needs of its citizenry still resonate today and serve as an exemplar for the continued value of the role of the public health nurse.

Historians often find it amazing that what has been written more than 100 years ago reflects the ideas of today. In Chapter 3, we see the need for school nurses reflected time and time again in urban and, even more so, in rural settings. The future of the country relies on the health of its young! So why not more school nurses? And, what is the role of the school nurse? As Mary Eckenrode Gibson notes, school nurses provide families the access to health care that they might not typically have. All children, especially those from particularly vulnerable populations, need the resources that a school nurse can provide. Gibson clearly lays out the statistics supporting this need, as well as the historical background of school nursing that reflects the challenges nurses faced in rural settings as they brought health care into the classroom. The role of the school nurse over the past 100 years provides a broad view of public health nursing that needs to be amplified. The author's rationale reflects upon how nurses work with others in an interprofessional and collaborative role that results in political advocacy for more school nurses.

In Section II, we see social and political issues raised with a world embroiled in war. Wartime raises questions about ethical behaviors as well as how nursing care continues amid destruction and despair. How do nurses carry on with the work of providing adequate nutrition, when doing so might mean sending the troops back to the war zone? Why did some nurses consent to government-sanctioned euthanasia and others did not? What lessons can we learn from these legal and ethical issues in our contemporary role development today? We often take for granted the nutrition needed to live, and we rarely see nourishment as part of a conversation about nursing during war or crisis. Yet, without proper nourishment, people will not heal, and any semblance of normalcy is lost.

In Chapter 4, Jane Brooks asks the reader to consider nursing under the duress caused by war—whether on the battlefield or in internment camps. Brooks considers nursing's role of ensuring an environment in which someone can heal, even at times when it means sending them back to a war zone when healed.

Brooks's discussion of the ethical dilemma, as well as the pragmatic role of providing nutrition, resonates with us today as nurses face the challenge to provide food to those in need—whether in our current war environments around the world, or in our urban and rural settings where hunger for many underserved populations exists as a daily reality. The chapter considers how wartime behaviors that include killing and maiming poise challenges to nursing's professional values that are dedicated to healing. As nurses today from across the world care for civilians and combatants in a variety of war zones, Brooks asks us to consider questions about nursing's political involvement in these conflicts. Brooks also asks that we look at the expertise that military nurses needed to ensure that the injured, diseased, and malnourished patients received adequate nutrition when that may not have been easily available. Nursing can be informed by this particular historical exemplar, and this chapter presents an opportunity to dialogue about this nursing role in the ever-present war zones of today.

In Chapter 5, historians Linda Shields and Susan Benedict address an often-hidden historical exemplar to demonstrate the ways in which nursing ethics and the state can sometimes conflict. In Nazi Germany, the edicts of the state and the ethics of the profession collided, profoundly affecting how some nurses treated those entrusted to their care.

Since the start of the American Nurses Association in 1896, nurses have discussed the moral and ethical ways to conduct oneself in practice and private life. A code of ethics was finally adopted in 1950 and continues to evolve today. Similarly, the International Council of Nurses that began in 1899 adopted an international code in 1953. These codes were developed as a direct response to the atrocities committed in World War II, but even before then semblances of codes existed in the United States and internationally, including laws that governed the way the state could influence health care professionals and their work. Nurses in Nazi Germany and other situations acted against these laws, and this continues to be an important issue for nurses today.

Nurses must reflect on their individual behavior and that of the profession (historically and currently) in which they took an oath to uphold the welfare of their patients, regardless of country or state. In this chapter, Shields and Benedict provide us with an exemplar from history where the professional ethics of nurses conflicted with governmental edicts. Some nurses succumbed to the alternative values espoused by the Nazi regime, whereas others stood fast to the ethical principles to which nursing subscribed. Shields and Benedict ask the reader to consider how they would have responded then and how they would respond now to some of the ethical dilemmas nurses face today—whether related to pro-life or pro-choice, euthanasia, determining organ donors, or prolonging life. History can inform these discussions and ultimately our decisions.

Section III highlights the years immediately following World War II, in which nurses were needed at home, new educational programs were established, and questions about the differentiation of the roles of the nurse were raised. As we see, these questions about whether nurses need to be educated at the university level, and whether that makes a difference in the practice of the nursing role, continue to be widely debated.

In Chapter 6, coeditor Kylie M. Smith writes with Geertje Boschma to address the development of mental health nursing as a clinical specialty, demonstrating the way in which this central component of human health has been subject to political and social forces often beyond its control. Yet nurses themselves were active in this time period, advocating for a distinct and independent role of the nurse as a therapeutic agent. This required the generation of advanced knowledge and educational programs, made possible by post–World War II concerns with social stability and the subsequent shift of attention and funding toward the mental health sciences. Increasing concerns with human and patient rights fed into the move toward deinstitutionalization, and the move to community-based mental health services required that nurses themselves develop new approaches to practice that relied on relationships with patients. The authors demonstrate that mental health nurses were capable of high-level theorizing and innovation, but that mental health continues to be a problematic area of practice linked to historical, political, and cultural attitudes toward mental illness itself.

April D. Matthias offers another view of nursing education as she explores the differentiation of practice and how the three educational pathways prepared nurses for practice. In Chapter 7, Matthias takes a close look at the failure of the nursing profession to define the practice role of each of the three pathways: diploma, associate degree, and baccalaureate degree. The different pathways all culminate in the same licensing exam and as a result nurses share the same practice role based on licensure and not on level of education. The nursing profession has grappled with this entry-into-practice issue almost since the inception of the Nightingale training schools. Contemporary efforts to advance the education of the nurse and to define the baccalaureate degree as the minimum educational preparation have been bolstered by evidence-based research citing a better patient outcome in hospitals with a higher percentage of baccalaureate-degree nurses (Aiken, Clark, & Chung, 2003; Aiken, Clark, & Sloane, 2002; Institute of Medicine [IOM], 2010). Matthias broadens the understanding of each entry level by including an examination of early programs: the Bellevue School of Nursing (1873) as the diploma case study, the University of Cincinnati

School for Nursing and Health (1916) as the bachelor of science in nursing (BSN) case study, and the Cooperative Research Project (CRP) in Junior and Community College Education for Nursing (1952), which resulted in the associate degree nurse (ADN) model for the education of nurses. Each pathway was developed with the intent of advancing the education of nurses and differentiating the practice role of each type of education. Although the pathway developments did succeed in advancing the education of some nurses, role differentiation did not occur. Matthias argues that the current "BSN in 10" efforts still do not address the lack of defined practice roles of the nursing workforce, and the lack of a phased plan to terminate diploma and associate-degree programs allows for the continued production of nurses from multiple program types. Her chapter informs the reader of the barriers to a single pathway into the profession, as well as past flawed strategies as we continue to advocate the baccalaureate degree as the minimal requirement for all nurses.

Following Matthias's chapter, a closer look at the history of the ADN is explored through the lens of preparing the educator. The educator role lies squarely within the purview of the professional nurse. Whether educating new nurses, new graduates, or patients and their families, teaching is inherent in this position. Yet rarely is this role examined from the perspective of how we educate nurses to fulfill this important function. In Chapter 8, coeditor of this book Annemarie McAllister uncovers a long-forgotten history of how nurse leaders at Teachers College, Columbia University in New York, the mecca for educating early nurse educators and administrators, developed a curriculum in the late 1950s specifically for the faculty role in the newly developed associate degree programs. McAllister provides us with an understanding of what the world was like following World War II, and why this country embraced the need for more education of all Americans, including nurses. With the rise of the community college–based associate degree programs in the early 1950s, the need for faculty in this college-based setting soared. Nurse leaders adapted to this challenge by developing systematic programs to educate the educators in associate degree programs. This author provides us a look at this important story in nursing that shows innovative ways that support nurses in their role as educators. Much can be learned from this past experience to meet the challenges of our nursing programs today.

In Section IV, we examine the volatile years of the Civil Rights and Women's Liberation movements, where we see the professional role of

the neonatal nurse develop, where nurses undertook extensive advocacy efforts to provide the best care for those with sickle cell anemia in
Canada, and nursing advocacy specifically for women's health care as
a civil right comes to our attention. Nurses continually address the ten-
sion that surrounds the perception of nursing as a profession. Today,
given the goals set out by a national agenda, such as found in the
Affordable Care Act and the IOM's report *The Future of Nursing: Leading
Change, Advancing Health* (IOM, 2010), nurses, the public, and legislators
in particular need greater clarity about this role. Nurses must be able
to practice to the fullest extent that their education prepares them to
perform. That means the professional role must be fully actualized
by those in nursing, as well as others. In Chapter 9, Briana Ralston
Smith addresses the ideas about nursing and the developing professional
role through the lens of caring for the very vulnerable population of
critically ill neonates. Through the work of these early pioneering nurses,
she establishes the ideas about what a profession is, and addresses the
conflicting views about such a profession. Using the newly developing
NICUs of the 1960s and 1970s, Ralston Smith shows how nurses honed
their knowledge and skills to provide the quality care that was so
needed. Nurses became central to the story about this emerging field
of practice, along with other relevant players, such as physicians who
typically receive the accolades. This raises the question of gender, and
broadens the discussion on how it affects the notion of professionalism. Ralston Smith establishes nursing as a profession in this chapter
and this in turn allows us to think about how we actualize this role in
all health care settings today.

In Chapter 10, Karen Flynn shows how nurses serve as advocates
for their patients, families, and communities. Early nursing leaders
knew they had the knowledge and skills to speak for others. Nurses
have a responsibility to advocate for all, regardless of race, class, ethnicity, gender, or illness. Flynn brings this to light in her chapter that
shows how one nurse, Lillie Johnson, advocated to help others, especially nurses, understand and care for those with sickle cell anemia—
an illness that did not get the attention that was so needed. Johnson led
a path advocating inclusion of this disorder in nursing school curricula,
in legislative debates, and in the minds of community activists. By
increasing awareness and engaging in dialogue, the outcomes for those
faced with this life-threatening disease improved.

In Chapter 11, Linda Tina Maldonado and Barbra Mann Wall contribute to the contemporary discussion about women's health. Women's

health care, while a private matter, needed the political advocacy of nurses in the public arena. Margaret Sanger, founder of Planned Parenthood, continually sought to challenge the laws that prohibited the distribution of birth control information during the first half of the 20th century. She started a clinic in Brooklyn, New York, where birth control information was distributed among women in the community who wanted to gain access. In this chapter, we see a history of nursing's engagement in community action, specifically directed at supporting women's health. The authors provide us with nursing's work with community coalitions that connect the many stakeholders interested in the rights of others. Social justice, civil rights, and access to health care, linked together, are all part of the advocacy role that nurses have engaged in the past, and continue to do so today. Read this chapter and consider the role nurses can play today as we address health care disparities while building a culture of health.

Qualified instructors may obtain access to an ancillary instructor's manual by e-mailing textbook@springerpub.com.

CONCLUSION

Nursing History for Contemporary Role Development offers an account of the historical development of some contemporary issues in nursing. These are not the only issues, and these chapters do not provide all the answers. Despite our efforts to explain it, history itself is not neat and concise and there are many ways to view historical phenomena. But a historical sensibility does show, as these authors illustrate, that contemporary nursing has evolved as a result of political, economic, and social forces particular to time and place. Using case studies from the past to highlight nurses' active participation in the development of their own practice and profession, we see the many ways in which nurses learned the work that was required to care for various populations. At times, nurses succeeded in bringing health care to those in need by advocating political and social change. At other times, nurses looked to educational reforms, such as university-based education versus hospital-based diploma training, to actualize their role. Negotiating the emergence of complex legal and ethical issues, nurses at times succumbed to political views that contradicted nursing's developing moral and ethical code. Yet nurses, through war and peacetime, continued to challenge the profession to raise its standards and address society's health care needs. Today's concerns for the vulnerable, the underserved, and the disparities that plague health care reform efforts continue to motivate the ever-changing (and hopefully improving) nature of nursing practice. The editors encourage readers to engage with all of the chapters, whether in order or not, so that they may continue the conversations that nurses started decades ago.

Sandra B. Lewenson
Annemarie McAllister
Kylie M. Smith

REFERENCES

Aiken, L., Clarke, S., Cheung, R., Sloane, D., & Silber, J. (2003). Education levels of hospital nurses and surgical patient mortality. *Journal of the American Medical Association, 290*(12), 1617–1623.

Aiken, L., Clarke, S., Sloane, D., Sochalski, J., & Silber, J. (2002). Hospital nurse staffing and patient mortality, nurse burnout, and job dissatisfaction. *Journal of the American Medical Association, 288,* 1987–1993.

D'Antonio, P., Connolly, C., Wall, B. M., Whelan, J. C., & Fairman, J. (2010). Histories of nursing: The power and the possibilities. *Nursing Outlook, 58*(4), 207–213.

Fairman, J., & D'Antonio, P. (2013). History counts: How history can help our understanding of health policy. *Nursing Outlook, 61,* 346–352.

Healthy People 2020. (2016). Determinants of health. Washington, DC: Office of Disease Prevention and Health Promotion. Retrieved from http://www.healthypeople.gov/2020/about/foundation-health-measures/Determinants-of-Health

Institute of Medicine (IOM). (2010). *The future of nursing: Leading change, advancing health*. Washington, DC: National Academies Press.

Lewenson, S. B. (2004). Integrating nursing history into the curriculum. *Journal of Professional Nursing, 20*(6), 374–380.

Lewenson, S. B., & McAllister, A. (2015). Historical method. Learning the historical method: Step by step. In M. de Chesnay (Ed.), *Nursing research using historical methods: Qualitative designs and methods in nursing* (pp. 1–21). New York, NY: Springer Publishing.

McAllister, M., John, T., & Gray, M. (2009). In my day: Using lessons from history, ritual and our elders to build professional identity. *Nurse Education in Practice, 9*(4), 277–283.

McAllister, A., & Lewenson, S. B. (2015). Inside track of doing historical research: My dissertation story. In M. de Chesnay (Ed.), *Nursing research using historical methods: Qualitative designs and methods in nursing* (pp. 41–58). New York, NY: Springer Publishing.

McAllister, M., Madsen, W., Godden, J., Greenhill, J., & Reed, R. (2010). Teaching nursing's history: A national survey of Australian schools of nursing, 2007–2008. *Nurse Education Today, 30*(4), 370–375.

Smith, K. M., Brown, A., & Crookes, P. A. (2015). History as reflective practice: A model for integrating historical studies into nurse education. *Collegian, 22*(3), 341–347.

Toman, C., & Thifault, M. C. (2012). Historical thinking and the shaping of nursing identity. *Nursing History Review, 20*(1), 184–204.

Wald, L. D. (1918a, May). *Address at Graduation Johns Hopkins Hospital.* Lillian Wald Papers (Writings & Speeches, Nurses & Nursing II, Reel 25, pp. 1–12). New York Public Library, New York, NY.

Wald, L. D. (1918b, March 5). *The woman voter should realize the relation of the visiting nurse to public health: The designer.* Lillian Wald Papers (Writings & Speeches, Voters & Voting, Reel 25, p. 1). New York Public Library, New York, NY.

Acknowledgments

Over the past 2 years, we three editors met on a regular basis to discuss the history of nursing and what it means for contemporary practice. We started with Skype meetings between New York and Wollongong in Australia—two of us finishing the day with our meeting, while the third was just starting hers. When Kylie moved to Atlanta, we were at least in the same time zone, and by meeting every month, and then every week, we completed our proposal; considered what to include; contacted our contributors; set up deadlines; invited Donna Avanecean, a doctor of nursing practice student, to work with us as our graduate assistant; and proceeded to embark on this journey of producing a book designed to bring our belief in the importance of nursing history into the world view of our students.

We owe a debt of gratitude to all the contributors who supported this project, and to our editors at Springer Publishing Company, Joseph Morita, who helped tame our original idea, and Rachel Landes, who helped whip the words into shape. We especially want to thank our families, friends, furkids, and colleagues who continually support the efforts of this writing team! Throughout the writing of this book, we endured transcontinental moves, weddings, births, deaths, and a lot of shopping. We continued in the face of life's events and became stronger editors and writers as a result.

This was a team effort right from the beginning. We shared our ideas, considered the ideas of others, and critiqued each other's work and those of our contributors. And without this great team, this book would not have come together. We started this journey because we believe that the nurses and students of today need to understand the paths their forebearers carved out. We want today's nurses and students to be as inspired and challenged as we are by that history. Every decision we made in the process of this book was made with them in mind, and they were as much a part of the team as we were.

One final acknowledgment must go to those institutions and organizations that support the inclusion of historical scholarship. Many thanks go to the leaders of the Mellon Foundation, the Barbara Bates Center for the Study of the History of Nursing, the Eleanor Crowder Bjoring Center for Nursing Historical Inquiry, and the American Association for the History of Nursing, to name a few, for creating the environment in which this work can flourish.

Section I: Late 19th and Early 20th Century

Chapter 1: Minority Nurses in Diverse Communities: Mary Elizabeth Tyler and the Whittier Centre in Early 20th-Century Philadelphia

J. MARGO BROOKS CARTHON

Because nurses make up the largest proportion of the health care workforce and work across virtually every health care and commu-nity-based setting, changing the demographic composition of nurses has the potential to effect changes in the face of health care in America.
(Institute of Medicine [IOM], 2011, p. 128)

Racial and ethnic minorities in the United States have endured long-standing health disparities. Minority populations on average experi-ence shorter life expectancies, higher rates of complications following surgery, and poorer clinical management of many conditions, includ-ing congestive heart failure, cancer, pain, hypertension, and diabetes (Carthon, Jarrin, Sloane, & Kutney-Lee, 2013; Hossain, Ahteshan, Salman, Jenson, & Calkins, 2013; National Center for Health Statistics, 2013). In addition, non-Whites are more likely to be unimmunized, lack preventive services, and use emergency departments (EDs) and hospi-tals for conditions that should not advance to ED or hospital visits if properly managed in primary care settings (Ginde, Espinola, & Camargo, 2008; McGlynn et al., 2003; Trivedi, Zaslavsky, Schneider, & Ayanian, 2005). Disparities in health outcomes often arise from com-plex factors, including higher rates of poverty, lower health literacy, and poorer quality in health care settings where minorities receive care (Howard, Sentell, & Gazmararian, 2006; Jha, Orav, & Epstein, 2011).

Efforts to reduce health disparities have taken the national spotlight in recent decades with many studies recommending that health inequities may be reduced through a focus on health care providers (Horner et al., 2004) and by increasing the number of nurses from underrepresented minority backgrounds (Institute of Medicine [IOM], 2011). A diverse health care workforce has long been linked to improvements in minority health outcomes (Grumbach & Mendoza, 2008), and there are many examples of the ways in which minority nurses have served as leaders in initiatives to improve population health for diverse communities (Carnegie, 1993; Carthon, 2011a). Despite these contributions, the numbers of nurses from diverse backgrounds remain relatively small. In 1910, the percentage of non-White nurses in the United States was 4% (D'Antonio & Whelan, 2009). By 1980, that percentage increased to just above 6% (Health Resources and Services Administration [HRSA], 2007). The most recent estimates, according to the 2008 National Sample Survey of Registered Nurses (NSSRN), revealed that nurses from underrepresented racial/ethnic backgrounds were 16.8% of the total RN population (HRSA, 2010). The composition of minority nurses stands in stark contrast to the proportion of minorities in the U.S. populace. According to the 2010 U.S. Census Bureau, minorities represent approximately 37% of the U.S. population but are projected to reach majority status within the next three decades (U.S. Census Bureau, 2010).[1]

The nursing workforce may face difficulties in meeting the cultural and linguistic demands of the 21st century given that its composition remains more than 80% White, and less than 5% of this workforce is proficient in a language other than English (Sullivan, 2004). Recent reports, including the IOM's (2011) *The Future of Nursing: Leading Change, Advancing Health* and Smedley, Smith, and Nelson's (2003) *Unequal Treatment: Confronting Racial and Ethnic Disparities in Health Care*, suggest increasing diversity in the health care workforce as a strategy to

---

1. This chapter employs the categories employed by the U.S. Census Bureau when referring to racial and ethnic "minorities" (Humes, Jones, & Ramirez, 2011), which identifies five racial categories: White, Black or African American, American Indian or Alaska Native, Asian, and Native Hawaiian or Other Pacific Islander and Hispanic, which is regarded as a separate category in which individuals can identify as a race and Hispanic.

reduce health disparities. Results from these studies suggest that a diverse health care workforce fosters better patient–provider communication, enhances patient satisfaction, increases access to care, and improves adherence to treatment plans (Meghani et al., 2009).

Examples of how nursing diversity has positively influenced population health may be found through a review of historical sources. The case study in this chapter presents an example of minority nurses working collaboratively with community members in an urban setting to address health disparities during the early 20th century. Many of the norms, values, and institutional infrastructures present in minority communities remain in place today. Thus, a fuller appreciation of the dynamic and reciprocal relationship between community members and minority health care providers can serve as a template for efforts to promote health in minority communities today (Carthon, 2011b).

BACKGROUND

Two landmark studies in the past decade by Smedley et al. (2003; *Unequal Treatment*) and Sullivan (2004; *Missing Persons: Minorities in the Health Professions*) noted a direct link between the shortage of minority health care providers and poorer health outcomes for minorities. In defining the need for diversity across health professions, both studies concluded that diversity not only stood to improve health outcomes of patients and families, but also to improve the cultural competence of health care systems.

Sullivan (2004) defined racial and ethnic diversity in the health care workforce as encompassing several key characteristics including:

(1) the representation of all racial and ethnic groups from the community served within a given health care agency, institution, or system; (2) the system-wide incorporation of diverse skills, talents, and ideas from those ethnic groups; and (3) the sharing of professional-development opportunities and resources, as well as responsibilities and power among all racial and ethnic groups and at all levels of a given agency, institution, or system. (pp. 13–14)

Increasing diversity in the health care workforce is viewed as one mechanism to increase cultural competence. Cultural competence is described as "a set of behaviors, attitudes, customs, policies, and resources that come together in a system, agency or among professionals to enable that system, agency or those professionals to work effectively in cross cultural situations" (Sullivan, 2004, p. 16). Increasing the pool of nurses from diverse backgrounds ensures that there are members of the health care team who are able to navigate, identify, and understand the cross-cultural challenges of diverse patients and families.

In today's health care marketplace, diverse individuals and families require health care that is patient centered and tailored to meet individual needs and expectations. Culture often plays an important role in the way health care is viewed and can play a significant role in the way that patients perceive health education and their willingness to use it. Culture is defined as an integrated pattern of shared beliefs and behaviors that include the language, thoughts, communications, actions, customs, beliefs, values, and institutions of racial, ethnic, religious, or social groups (Office of Minority Health, 2000). Many minority populations find it important that providers have a deep understanding of their cultural beliefs and preferences surrounding health care. Some minority populations prefer clinicians who speak the same language or who share or understand similar values (Cooper & Powe, 2004). Higher ratings of satisfaction are noted, for example, among Spanish-speaking, Chinese, and Vietnamese patients when they are cared for by language-concordant providers (Betancourt, Green Carrillo, & Ananeh-Firempong, 2003; Ngo-Metzger et al., 2007). Similarly, when physicians employ a participatory and inclusive style of decision making, African American patients report more satisfaction with care (Betancourt et al., 2003). The incorporation of nonconventional healing systems, such as complementary and alternative medicine (CAM), may be important to other communities (O'Connor, 1995). Cultural competence is an important principle that underlies interactions between patient, provider, and systems. Health care professionals who understand or share the cultural preferences of their patients are often well positioned to work with diverse communities.

In addition to enhancing cultural competence, health professionals from underrepresented backgrounds bring diverse perspectives and are more likely to work in underserved communities (Komaromy et al., 1996). Health care providers from diverse backgrounds may also be able to mitigate feelings of alienation and frustration expressed by members of minority communities. Many minorities have experienced overt discrimination or bias from health care systems and providers (LaVeist, Nickerson, & Bowie, 2000). These experiences have led to mistrust and, in some instances, avoidance of health care services. Studies suggest that increasing the diversity of the health care workforce can improve quality of care for minorities as patients build trust and rapport with providers.

CASE STUDY: Nurses From Diverse Backgrounds Play Important Roles in Caring for the Needs of the Underserved

An example of the work of minority nurses was evident during the tuberculosis (TB) crisis in Philadelphia, Pennsylvania, at the turn of the 20th century. Like many large, Northern cities, Philadelphia had an increasingly diverse population as European immigrants and Blacks from the South arrived seeking jobs and opportunity. A housing shortage, poor sanitation, and a lack of proper ventilation led to high infant and maternal mortality rates. Mortality rates were particularly high among poor Blacks; for example, in 1900 Philadelphia, Black residents had two to three times more deaths due to TB than did White residents (Carthon, 2011a). Few people could afford medical services; others chose to remain in their homes during illness out of fear of hospitals or a preference for traditional healing methods. Many hospitals had policies that refused care to Blacks or offered care in segregated wards (Rice & Jones, 1994).

Overwhelmed by the city's needs, health officials were often assisted by philanthropic charities that provided health services and social resources (Carthon, 2011b). The Whittier Centre, a local charity founded in 1912, was an example of a philanthropic association organized to address community health and housing concerns. In May 1913, members of the Whittier Centre met to discuss suitable ways to reduce the effects of TB, which was ravaging the Black community (Figure 1.1).

(continued)

CASE STUDY: Nurses From Diverse Backgrounds Play Important Roles in Caring for the Needs of the Underserved *(continued)*

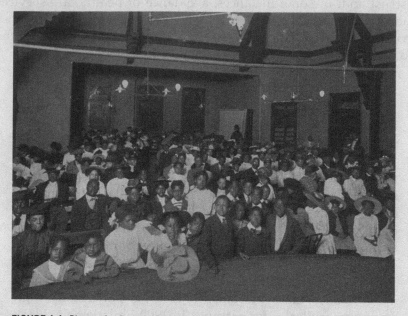

FIGURE 1.1 Photo of a Coal Club Meeting.

Source: Starr Centre Annual Report. (1906). Starr Centre Association Collection, Barbara Bates Center for the Study of the History of Nursing, School of Nursing. University of Pennsylvania, Philadelphia, PA.

Much of the excessive illness among Black residents was linked to factors such as racism, poverty, and inadequate housing (Wright, 1935). In addition, local hospitals and private sanitariums often placed restrictions on admitting Black patients (McBride, 1989). Those that did admit Blacks often suffered from overcrowding and disrepair (Committee on Municipal Charities of Philadelphia, 1913). During the meeting, a White physician and TB expert, Dr. Henry Landis, voiced his concerns over the excessive TB deaths among Black Philadelphians and proposed hiring a Black nurse as a strategy to encourage Black residents to seek help at the local TB clinic. Landis expressed the advantages of this proposition, saying, "to really get behind

(continued)

CASE STUDY: Nurses From Diverse Backgrounds Play Important Roles in Caring for the Needs of the Underserved *(continued)*

the scenes" of health conditions in Black homes it would require a person of the same race (Whittier Centre, 1913, p. 1). According to Landis, a Black nurse could more easily gain patients' confidence and dispel any fears or superstitions regarding illness that might prevent Blacks from seeking care. Once hired, her duties would be that of a visiting nurse, sanitary inspector, and social worker. She was expected to not only work in the community, she was also to live in the district and establish a "neighborhood house" where she would serve as a liaison between community members and the Whittier Centre's health objectives.

The Whittier Centre's proposal to hire a Black nurse was at the time regarded as a novel experiment. Up until this point, there is little evidence to suggest that Black clinicians held prominent positions in the anti-TB campaign in Philadelphia (Landis, 1923; Mossell, 1923). At this meeting, however, the members of the Whittier Centre board of directors took a step away from tradition and on that day agreed to provide the salary of $65 per month to hire its first Black nurse—Mary Elizabeth Tyler (Figure 1.2).

Tyler began her new position on February 1, 1914, providing services to the Henry Phipps Institute. The Henry Phipps Institute was established in 1903 as the nation's first endowed center for research and clinical campaigns to prevent and eradicate TB (Bates, 1992; McBride, 1987). As a member of the Henry Phipps Institute staff, Tyler's job included locating Black residents suspected of having TB, and then referring them to the Phipps Clinic for treatment. Prior to her arrival, it was well known that few Blacks sought care for TB despite the Phipps Clinic's location in the heart of the city's historical Black district (Pitts Mosely, 1996).

Tyler's education and past professional experience had prepared her well for her new assignment. As a graduate of Freedman's Hospital Training School in Washington, DC, she

(continued)

CASE STUDY: Nurses From Diverse Backgrounds Play Important Roles in Caring for the Needs of the Underserved (continued)

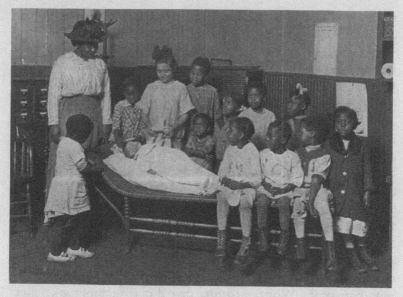

FIGURE 1.2 Whittier Centre, "Annual Report," 1915.

Source: Reprinted with the permission of the Urban Archives, Temple University Libraries.

was the recipient of a premier education. After graduation, she worked as a private duty nurse in Northampton, Massachusetts, and then as a resident nurse and instructor of physiology and hygiene at Alabama A&M University, Normal, Alabama. In 1906, she accepted a position as the first Black visiting nurse of the Henry Street Settlement in New York City (Pitts Mosely, 1996). During her time as a public health nurse in New York, she worked among poor Black and immigrant families with health concerns similar to those that she would face once arriving in Philadelphia.

Tyler's first year in Philadelphia was spent providing home care to 327 families that were intimately affiliated with the Whittier Centre. The number of persons in these families totaled well over 1,000 (Whittier Centre, 1914). Of those members

(continued)

CASE STUDY: Nurses From Diverse Backgrounds Play Important Roles in Caring for the Needs of the Underserved *(continued)*

visited, 12% were suspected of having TB and were sub-sequently referred to the hospital or clinic for treatment. After receiving fair treatment at the TB clinic, patients then referred friends and family to the clinic for similar care. In the first year of her work in Philadelphia, more than 12 times the number of Black patients visited the clinic than had during the first 11 years of the Henry Phipps Institute's history. So effective were these efforts that, within 6 months of Tyler's hire, another Black nurse, Cora Johnson, was added to the Henry Phipps Institute staff. Later that same year, a Black physician, Henry Minton, joined to oversee the care of Black patients at the dispensary. Their salaries were paid by the Philadelphia Committee of the Pennsylvania Society for the Study of Tuberculosis and the Pennsylvania State Department of Health (Whittier Centre, 1915).

Instrumental to Tyler's success was her ability to extend her nursing care to areas beyond the boundaries of health. During her home visits, Tyler first built a strong rapport with neighborhood families and then inquired about their health conditions and their housing and economic concerns. In her first year, Tyler found that nearly 62% of the families visited required medical or social services (Whittier Centre, 1915). For Tyler, this meant offering advice, providing lectures on health, making referrals to other civic agencies, or recommending treatment at the Henry Phipps Institute (Figure 1.3). As a result, Tyler was recognized as an important community resource—working closely with families, civic leaders, and other health professionals.

Tyler was also a health educator and, during her first year in Philadelphia, helped to organize three "Little Mothers' Clubs" in the neighborhood. As members of the clubs, girls received lessons on hygiene, breastfeeding, and childcare, which were used as a means to reduce infant mortality in the city. In addition to these activities, Tyler helped to organize a club composed of

(continued)

CASE STUDY: Nurses From Diverse Backgrounds Play Important Roles in Caring for the Needs of the Underserved *(continued)*

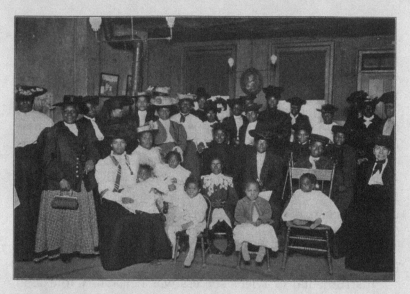

FIGURE 1.3 Tyler Meets with Members of Community Civic Associations.

Source: Starr Centre Annual Report. (1911). Starr Centre Association Collection, Barbara Bates Center for the Study of the History of Nursing, School of Nursing. University of Pennsylvania, Philadelphia, PA.

women in the immediate neighborhood who desired to address community issues (Whittier Centre, 1915). The work of this club, along with the other activities of the Whittier Centre, solidified Tyler's base and allowed her to introduce health promotion initiatives in concert with other community-building efforts. Over the decade following her hire, the Whittier Centre's involvement with community health grew to include the establishment of several health centers, including a prenatal clinic, well-baby clinics, and home supervision. By 1927, the staff of Black clinicians, then known as the Negro Health Bureau, grew from one nurse to 10 and from one physician to 12 (Landis, 1927).

DISCUSSION AND CONCLUSION

The changing face of the U.S. populace requires a health care system that is responsive to the beliefs and values of diverse populations. Increasing diversity in nursing offers opportunities for health professionals from underrepresented backgrounds to serve in instrumental roles to meet the needs of diverse populations. Nurses currently make up the largest proportion of health care professionals in the United States and have a long history of providing care to the underserved (Carthon, 2011a, 2011b). As a minority nurse, Elizabeth Tyler was in a unique position. She was aware of the social, political, and economic factors effecting Black community members and used this knowledge to create relationships while addressing the most pressing needs of her patient population. Tyler's cultural affinity with Black community residents allowed her to use this shared background to garner trust, which permitted her to introduce health-promoting behaviors. The addition of Tyler to the anti-TB campaign represents an example of diversity in action.

Embracing diversity among health care professionals and valuing differences among patients is a core feature of the nursing profession that was reflected in nursing's past and remains relevant today. The American Nurses Association's (ANA, 2010) edition of *Nursing's Social Policy Statement: The Essence of the Profession* notes that nurses in their roles as caregivers and advocates are required to provide caring relationships with the potential to heal, be attuned to the human response to illness within the context of social and physical environments, and influence public policy to promote social justice (ANA, 2010). These tenets of the nursing profession define the role of a nurse as one who responds to the objective and subjective concerns of patients, and then integrates care management goals with the values and preferences of patients. Elizabeth Tyler demonstrated these characteristics more than a century ago as a community nurse working in a minority community, yet *all* nurses, irrespective of racial and ethnic affiliations, can serve as an "Elizabeth Tyler" in their individual clinical settings by advocating for patient-centered, culturally competent care for patients and family members.

ACTIVITIES FOR TEACHING AND LEARNING

Although history teaches many lessons about how diverse nurses helped to improve patient and community outcomes, it is important for students to be able to "connect the dots" between the inclusion of minorities in nursing historically and with today's concerns related to health disparities. Similarly, cultural competence and understanding the impact of culture on views of health are not skills that only minority nurses should possess. Some questions for students to consider:

1. Would a public health initiative similar to the one discussed in this chapter be possible today?
2. What would the benefits be for having greater diversity in the nursing workforce today?
3. Should students be able to discuss the value of cultural competence for all nurses?
4. What skills will you need to gain as a nurse in order to work with diverse communities?

REFERENCES

American Nurses Association. (2010). *Nursing's social policy statement: The essence of the profession*. Silver Spring, MD: Nursesbooks.org.

Bates, B. (1992). *Bargaining for life: A social history of tuberculosis, 1876–1939*. Philadelphia: University of Pennsylvania Press.

Betancourt, J. R., Green, A. R., Carrillo, J. E., & Ananeh-Firempong, O., II. (2003). Defining cultural competence: A practical framework for addressing racial/ethnic disparities in health and health care. *Public Health Reports, 118*(4), 293.

Carnegie, M. E. (1993). *The path we tread: Blacks in nursing worldwide, 1954–1990*. Sudbury, MA: Jones & Bartlett.

Carthon, B. J., Jarrin, O., Sloane, D., & Kutney-Lee, A. (2013). Variations in postoperative complications according to race, ethnicity, and sex in older adults. *Journal of the American Geriatrics Society, 61*(9), 1499–1507.

Carthon, M. B. (2011a). Life and death in Philadelphia's Black Belt: A tale of an urban tuberculosis campaign, 1900–1930. *Nursing History Review, 19*, 29.

Carthon, M. B. (2011b). Making ends meet: Community networks and health promotion among Blacks in the city of Brotherly Love. *American Journal of Public Health, 101*(8), 1392–1401.

Committee on Municipal Charities of Philadelphia. (1913). *The report of the subcommittee on Tuberculosis.* Philadelphia, PA. Retrieved from the Temple University Urban Archives.

Cooper, L. A., & Powe, N. R. (2004). Disparities in patient experiences, health care processes, and outcomes: The role of patient-provider racial, ethnic, and language concordance. New York, NY: Commonwealth Fund. Retrieved from http://www.commonwealthfund.org/programs/minority/cooper_raceconcordance_753.pdf

D'Antonio, P., & Whelan, J. C. (2009). Counting nurses: The power of historical census data. *Journal of Clinical Nursing, 18*(19), 2717–2724.

Ginde, A. A., Espinola, J. A., & Camargo, C. A. (2008). Improved overall trends but persistent racial disparities in emergency department visits for acute asthma, 1993–2005. *Journal of Allergy and Clinical Immunology, 122*(2), 313–318.

Grumbach, K., & Mendoza, R. (2008). Disparities in human resources: Addressing the lack of diversity in the health professions. *Health Affairs, 27*(2), 413–422.

Health Resources and Services Administration. (2007). The registered nurse population: Findings from the 2004 National Sample Survey of Registered Nurses. Retrieved from http://bhpr.hrsa.gov/healthworkforce/rnsurveys/rnsurvey2004.pdf

Health Resources and Services Administration. (2010). The registered nurse population: Findings from the 2008 National Sample Survey of Registered Nurses. Retrieved from http://bhpr.hrsa.gov/healthworkforce/rnsurveys/rnsurveyfinal.pdf

Horner, R. D., Salazar, W., Geiger, H. J., Bullock, K., Corbie-Smith, G., Cornog, M., & Flores, G. (2004). Changing healthcare professionals' behaviors to eliminate disparities in healthcare: What do we know? How might we proceed? *The American Journal of Managed Care, 10,* SP12-9.

Hossain, A. W. A., Ahteshan, M. W., Salman, G. A., Jenson, R., & Calkins, C. F. (2013). Healthcare access and disparities in chronic medical conditions in urban populations. *Southern Medical Journal, 106*(4), 246–254.

Howard, D. H., Sentell, T., & Gazmararian, J. A. (2006). Impact of health literacy on socioeconomic and racial differences in health in an elderly population. *Journal of General Internal Medicine, 21*(8), 857–861.

Humes, K. R., Jones, N. A., & Ramirez, R. R. (2011). *Overview of race and Hispanic origin: 2010*. Washington, DC: U.S. Census Bureau. Retrieved from www .census.gov/prod/cen2010/briefs/c2010br-02.pdf

Institute of Medicine. (2010). The future of nursing: Leading change, advancing health. Retrieved from http://www.nationalacademies.org/hmd/ Reports/2010/The-Future-of-Nursing-Leading-Change-Advancing -Health.aspx

Jha, A. K., Orav, E. J., & Epstein, A. M. (2011). Low-quality, high-cost hospitals, mainly in the South, care for sharply higher shares of elderly black, Hispanic, and Medicaid patients. *Health Affairs, 30*(10), 1904–1911.

Komaromy, M., Grumbach, K., Drake, M., Vranizan, K., Lurie, N., Keane, D., & Bindman, A. B. (1996). The role of black and Hispanic physicians in providing health care for underserved populations. *New England Journal of Medicine, 334*(20), 1305–1310.

Landis, H. R. M. (1923). *A report of the tuberculosis problem and the Negro*. Philadelphia, PA: Henry Phipps Institute.

Landis, H. R. M. (1927). *The work of the Whittier Centre*. Philadelphia, PA: Philadelphia Housing Association.

LaVeist, T. A., Nickerson, K. J., & Bowie, J. V. (2000). Attitudes about racism, medical mistrust, and satisfaction with care among African American and white cardiac patients. *Medical Care Research and Review, 57*(Suppl. 4), 146–161.

McBride, D. (1987). The Henry Phipps Institute, 1903–1937: Pioneering tuberculosis work with an urban minority. *Bulletin of the History of Medicine, 61*(1), 78.

McBride, D. (1989). *Integrating the city of medicine; Blacks in Philadelphia healthcare, 1910-1965*. Philadelphia, PA: Temple University Press.

McGlynn, E. A., Asch, S. E., Adams, J., Keesey, J., Hicks, J., DeCristofaro, A., & Kerr, E. A. (2003). The quality of health care delivered to adults in the United States. *New England Journal of Medicine, 348*, 2635–2645.

Meghani, S. H., Brooks, J. M., Gipson-Jones, T., Waite, R., Whitfield-Harris, L., & Deatrick, J. (2009). Patient–provider race-concordance: Does it matter in improving minority patients' health outcomes? *Ethnicity & Health, 14*(1), 107–130.

Mossell, S. T. (1923). *A study of the Negro tuberculosis problem in Philadelphia*. Philadelphia, PA: Henry Phipps Institute.

National Center for Health Statistics. (2013). Deaths: Final data for 2013. Retrieved from http://www.cdc.gov/nchs/data/nvsr/nvsr64/nvsr64_02 .pdf

Ngo-Metzger, Q., Sorkin, D. H., Phillips, R. S., Greenfield, S., Massagli, M. P., Clarridge, B., & Kaplan, S. H. (2007). Providing high-quality care for limited English proficient patients: The importance of language concordance and interpreter use. *Journal of General Internal Medicine, 22*(2), 324–330.

O'Connor, B. B. (1995). *Healing traditions: Alternative medicine and the health professions.* Philadelphia: University of Pennsylvania Press.

Office of Minority Health. (2000). *Assuring cultural competence in health care: Recommendations for national standards and outcomes-focused research agenda.* Washington, DC: U.S. Department of Health and Human Services.

Pitts Mosely, M. O. (1996). Satisfied to carry the bag: Three black community health nurses' contributions to health reform, 1900–1937. *Nursing History Review, 4,* 65–82.

Rice, M. F., & Jones, W. (1994). *Public policy and the black hospital: From slavery to segregation to integration.* Westport, CT: Greenwood Publishing Group.

Smedley, B. D., Smith, A. Y., & Nelson, A. R. (2003). Unequal treatment: Confronting racial and ethnic disparities in health care. Washington, DC: Institute of Medicine.

Starr Centre Annual Report. (1906). Starr Centre Association Collection. Barbara Bates Center for the Study of the History of Nursing, School of Nursing. University of Pennsylvania, Philadelphia, PA.

Starr Centre Annual Report. (1911). Starr Centre Association Collection. Barbara Bates Center for the Study of the History of Nursing, School of Nursing, University of Pennsylvania, Philadelphia, PA

Sullivan, L. W. (2004). *Missing persons: Minorities in the health professions, a report of the Sullivan Commission on Diversity in the Healthcare Workforce.* Alexandria, VA: The Sullivan Alliance to Transform the Health Professions.

Trivedi, A. N., Zaslavsky, A. M., Schneider, E. C., & Ayanian, J. Z. (2005). Trends in the quality of care and racial disparities in Medicare managed care. *New England Journal of Medicine, 353*(7), 692–700.

U.S. Census Bureau. (2010). Overview of race and Hispanic origin. Retrieved from http://www.census.gov/prod/cen2010/briefs/c2010br-02.pdf

Whittier Centre. (1913). *Executive board meeting minutes.* Wharton Center Collection, University Libraries, Temple University, Philadelphia, PA.

Whittier Centre. (1914). *Whittier Centre annual report.* Temple University Libraries Urban Archives. Philadelphia, PA, 4–6.

Whittier Centre. (1915). *Whittier Centre annual report.* Philadelphia, PA, 3, 6.

Wright, L. T. (1935, January). Health problems of the Negro. *Interracial Review,* 8, 6–8.

Chapter 2: The Origins of Public Health Nursing: Meeting the Health Needs of Small Town America

SANDRA B. LEWENSON

The flowering of visiting nursing into a public health service requires some historical background to set it in its proper perspective, especially as its destiny is to share in the coming stages of a vast medical and scientific advance of world-wide extent.

(Dock & Stewart, 1931, p. 299)

Read any newspaper and you find public health issues front and center. For example, the recent outbreak of measles in the United States has led public health professionals, nurses included, to reflect on what this means in terms of health for children and families (Turkewitz & Cave, 2015). Another example appeared in a *New York Times* Op-Ed written by a physician who wrote about bringing back house calls for physicians (Jauhar, 2015). Although his idea was a good one, he omitted the long-standing role of public health nurses who have worked in the community throughout the past century and into today. Nurse historian Jean Whelan (2015) responded to Jauhar's (2015) comments by bringing to the public's attention nurses' historical role of providing home care within the community. Whelan blogged, "Quite simply, the burden of delivering care to home-bound patients and the hard work of preventing hospital readmittance has always fallen on nurses' shoulders" (n.p.).

These articles and others like them raise questions about the contemporary role nurses play in public health. Public health nurses address the core functions of "public health" that the Institute of Medicine

(IOM, 1988) identifies as "assessment, policy development, and assurance." Public health nurses engage in these core functions by participating in early identification of health problems, by participating in the development of policies based on evidence, and by ensuring that the public receives access to health services through public or private means (Truglio-Londrigan & Lewenson, 2013). In the United States, these three core functions are part of the government's policy as outlined in Healthy People 2020 that lays out an agenda for a healthier nation. Public health nurses work toward meeting the overarching goals of Healthy People 2020, which include attaining quality health care, achieving health equity, eliminating health disparities among vulnerable populations, creating social and physical environments that promote health for all, and promoting quality of life, healthy development, and health behaviors (U.S. Department of Health and Human Services [DHHS], 2010). The interaction of these determinants of health means that public health nurses must address the physical and social environment where people live, work, and play (Hassmiller, 2017); and they must take into account the individual behaviors and available health services, as well as biology and genetics of populations that affect achieving the goals laid out in Healthy People 2020.

In the United States, a country that ranks 26th in the world in life expectancy, public health nurses must participate in creating a culture of health that leads to better health outcomes (Hassmiller, 2017). Whether it be exercise programs for the elderly in the community, healthy food choices in schools, or smoke cessation programs for adults, public health nurses must collaborate with others in the public and private arena to meet these goals. The Robert Wood Johnson Foundation (RWJF) believes that building a culture of health "means shifting the values—and actions—of this country so that healthy decisions become part of everything Americans do" (Hassmiller, 2017, pp. 41–42). Public health nurses can play a role in this cultural shift within a broad primary health care framework that relies on collaboration, community activism, interprofessional relationships, shared decision making, and evidence-based practice initiatives.

This chapter explores public health nursing within a larger primary health care framework demonstrating how public health nursing evolved over time to meet the needs of the public. It defines the terms used in this discussion, explores the evolution of public health nursing in the United States, and presents a historical case study highlighting an early 20th-century experiment in providing public health nursing to rural communities. The American Red Cross began a rural public health nursing service in 1912, which became known as the Town and Country Nursing Service. It lasted until 1948 when other public and private public health agencies assumed this role. This chapter shows how the town of Red Hook, a rural community in upstate New York, affiliated with the Town and Country Nursing Service between the years 1915 and 1917, demonstrating how public health nurses and community activists assembled resources to ensure a healthier community.

Primary health care, public health, and *primary care* are terms that are used interchangeably. Yet, understanding the distinction between and among the terms is crucial, especially when looking at policy decisions being made in regard to care and reimbursement for that care (DeVille & Novick, 2011, p. 106; Lewenson & Truglio-Londrigan, 2017; Truglio-Londrigan, Singleton, Lewenson, & Lopez, 2013). Primary health care was first defined by the World Health Organization (WHO) in the 1978 Declaration of Alma-Ata. Basic tenets included the idea that health was viewed as a basic human right; that multiple disciplines and stakeholders needed to be involved to ensure health for all; and that all stakeholders needed to be engaged participants in the provision of health care both individually and collectively (Truglio-Londrigan et al., 2013). Today, the term primary health care reflects "a broader philosophical and holistic approach to health care" (Lewenson & Truglio-Londrigan, 2017, p. xii). The building of a culture of health where people live, work, and play provides us an example of primary health care.

Public health nursing was defined in 2013 by the American Public Health Association (2013) as "the practice of promoting and protecting the health of populations using knowledge from nursing, social, and public health sciences" (n.p.). Public health nursing fits within the philosophical paradigm of primary health care that is synergistic with the goals of Healthy People 2020 and the effort to build a culture of health. Greenhalgh (2007) refers to public health as a "cousin" of primary health care (p. xi) where public health nursing uses a primary care (point of service) perspective, as well as a population-based focus (Lewenson & Truglio-Londrigan, 2017).[1] Primary care typically focuses on the one-to-one relationship between the provider and the patient. Primary care reflects, for example, on the nurse practitioner's, midwife's, or physician's

---

1. For a more complete discussion of the evolution of the definitions of public health nursing, see Lewenson (2013).

direct point-of-care service model, where care is rendered to a specific individual within a larger population.

BACKGROUND

Florence Nightingale, the noted creator of what became known as the Modern Nursing Movement, shared her views of community health at the 1893 World's Fair exposition in Chicago. It was at this international exposition that the American Society of Superintendents of Training Schools for Nurses started. This organization became known as the National League of Nursing Education (NLNE) in 1912 and renamed the National League for Nursing (NLN) in 1952. Nightingale (1893/1949) spoke at that meeting about health visitors in the community, saying that "The health of the unity is the health of community. Unless you have the health of the unity there is no community health" (p. 35). A healthy society, Nightingale reflected, relied on a unified nursing presence to ensure the public's health. A few years later, influenced by Nightingale's words, the noted public health nursing leader in the United States, Lillian Wald (Figure 2.1), expanded on Nightingale's term, "health visitor," by coining the term "public health nurse." Wald experienced the need firsthand when providing nursing services to the immigrant poor on the Lower East Side of New York City. Noted for starting the Henry Street Settlement in 1893, Wald gave us a meaningful demonstration of public health nursing. She, along with other public health nurses, moved into the house on Henry Street and lived within the community in which they provided nursing and social services (Buhler-Wilkerson, 1993; Keeling & Lewenson, 2013).

The plight of the urban poor, especially the immigrants that flooded the streets of New York City in the late 19th and early 20th century, coincided with nursing's efforts to professionalize nursing. During this period, nursing schools opened in hospitals throughout the United States where students provided an inexpensive form of labor. Upon graduation, nurses turned to private duty or public health nursing to earn a living. Wald's ideas at the Henry Street Settlement attracted many to public health nursing. The nurses at the Henry Street Settlement (which later became the Visiting Nurse Service of New York) offered a wide array of nursing services in the community. Nurses cared for the sick in their homes, taught mothers how to keep their families healthy, advocated for parks in the community, sought legislation to improve

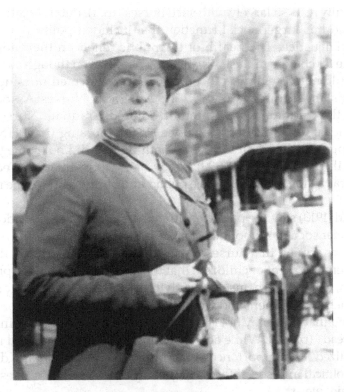

FIGURE 2.1 Lillian Wald.
Courtesy of the Visiting Nurse Service of New York.

living and work environments, and engaged in school nursing. To be effective in this expanded role, public health nurses needed additional coursework in areas, such as social services, rural sanitation, and the social sciences. By 1912, Teachers College (TC) of Columbia University in New York offered coursework that became a postgraduate requirement for public health nurses.

Political advocacy became central to the role of public health nurses in the early 20th century. Public health nurses such as Wald linked health care with legislative reforms and participated in efforts to improve housing, education, and environments for those living, working, and playing in the community. Wald (1918a) eloquently wrote that "women should support with their political influence the taxation and legislation which are needed for the establishment and the maintenance of visiting and public health nurses since the health of the community rests so largely with such nurses" (p. 1). Public health nurses embraced this larger social function that included political advocacy and social justice. The health of the public relied on their ability to advocate for change in the laws affecting health even though as women they could not vote. It was through the newly formed nursing organizations, including the NLNE, the American Nurses Association (ANA), the National Association of Colored Graduate Nurses, and the National Organization for Public Health Nursing (NOPHN), that nurses pursued the right to vote, something that did not come to fruition until 1920 (Lewenson, 1993). Lobbying for the right to vote equated to advocating for the health of the public, and became part of the nurse's role.

Wald (1913) saw the public health nurse's role as one that addresses the broader social and political concerns affecting the determinants of health. She argued that nurses "carry the obligation to prevent the premature employment of children, that they may conserve their physical strength; to identify themselves with the movements for the protection of the men and women who work, that dangers may be removed from them, and that they may not risk health or life itself while earning their daily bread" (p. 925). While acknowledging that all nurses had not yet "crystallized" the importance of their role, she saw that many did join in the political and social forces of the day. Public health nurses, Wald (1913) said, were

> educating the people, translating into simple terms the message of the expert and the scientist. The visiting nurses throughout the country have been inspired to dignify and to lay true values upon their service, coveting for themselves the privilege of relieving pain, and linking with that century-cherished prerogative of women, the new note of education and civic duty. (p. 925)

Nurses needed to understand and participate in the campaigns that sought a healthier society, such as serving on boards of sanitary control and working with schools and organizations that supported the health of the poor and middle class. Wald (1913) optimistically called upon the nursing organizations to stand together as a

> symbol of a universal sisterhood, dedicated to the service of their country through its people, young and old, rich and

poor, in institutions and in their homes, a circle unbroken until poverty and preventable disease shall be eliminated and the perfect civilization realized. (p. 926)

CASE STUDY: The American Red Cross Town and Country

Wald's vision to improve the health of the public expanded beyond the borders of urban centers. She recognized that those living in more rural towns and small cities required the same, if not more, kinds of health care services than those living in urban environments. Those living in more rural settings typically lacked sufficient numbers of health care providers who worked in larger cities. Distance between towns, especially in mountainous regions, and poor road conditions contributed to the lack of sufficient providers—both physicians and nurses—in these rural settings. Wald suggested that the American Red Cross (Figure 2.2), an organization that typically provided services during disasters either man-made or natural, could provide the national structure to reach small towns and communities throughout the United States (Buhler-Wilkerson, 1993; Dock, Pickett, Clement, Fox, & Van Meter, 1922; Lewenson, 2015).

By 1912, Wald had convinced the American Red Cross to support her vision to provide qualified public health nurses in rural towns and communities. In collaboration with the Rockefeller Foundation, wealthy philanthropists, and nursing leaders, the Town and Country Nursing Service officially began on November 12, 1912. Public health nursing leader Fannie Clement was appointed superintendent of this new service, and she served in this capacity until she moved into other Red Cross roles in Europe during World War I (Dock et al., 1922; Wald, 1921).

Fannie Clement was a 1903 graduate of Smith College and later a graduate of the Boston City Hospital Training School for Nurses (Kernodle, 1949, p. 73). She led the first few years of the Town and Country Nursing Service and worked with communities interested in affiliating with this rural nursing service. Each town that wanted a Town and Country public health

(continued)

CASE STUDY: The American Red Cross Town and Country *(continued)*

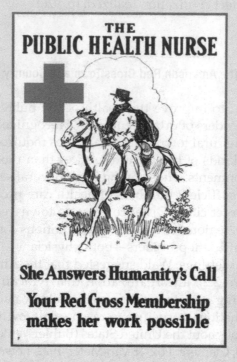

FIGURE 2.2 Poster advertising the American Red Cross Town and Country Nursing Service.

Courtesy of the American Red Cross.

nurse needed to complete an application asking for information about the town's health needs, its ability to pay the salary of the public health nurse, and the identification of other health care providers and interested stakeholders (e.g., physicians, school boards, church boards, pharmacists). Civic-minded women and men reached out to the Town and Country Nursing Service seeking help in establishing a visiting nursing service for their community much like the ones found in cities. Clement assured these applicants that they would receive an educated rural public health nurse skilled in establishing an appropriate nursing service within that town. In some communities that

(continued)

CASE STUDY: The American Red Cross Town and Country *(continued)*

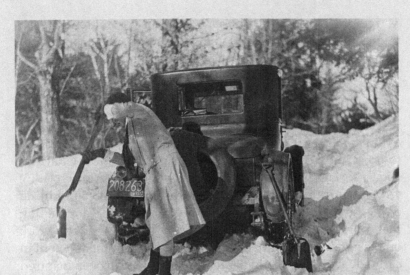

FIGURE 2.3 Rural public health nurse digging out her car from the snow, 1927.
Courtesy of the American Red Cross.

might mean providing a public health nurse who visited the
school, or who gave health talks to a church group, or who would
care for the sick in their homes (Figure 2.3).

The Red Hook Nursing Service Affiliates With the Town and Country

In 1915, Mary Gerard Lewis wrote to Clement for advice about
starting a rural visiting nursing service in her town of Red Hook
located in Dutchess County, New York. Lewis was the secretary
of the Red Hook nursing advisory committee that sought affiliation with the Town and Country Nursing Service. The membership of this committee represented a wide array of citizens
interested in the health care of the community. A wealthy
philanthropist and early supporter of professional nursing,

(continued)

CASE STUDY: The American Red Cross Town and Country *(continued)*

Margaret Chanler Aldrich, served on this committee. Aldrich frequently expressed her ideas in local newspapers, encouraging her fellow citizens to support the effort to affiliate with the Town and Country Nursing Service. She wrote about the appalling health care conditions in this rural county and the need for each resident to subscribe at least one dollar a year to hire a Red Cross Town and Country nurse. The need for the services of a rural public health nurse was clearly identified in a 1912 door-to-door study conducted in Dutchess County (State Charities Aid Association, 1915). Based on these findings, Aldrich (1916) wrote that unless the community was committed to fighting disease and hiring a nurse, the county would lag behind, noting that "our doctors cannot be our nurses" (n.p.). Aldrich's work on the nursing committee was preceded by her engagement in early advocacy-type activities for nursing. She had been inspired to take an interest in nursing by her great aunt, Julia Ward Howe, who was active in the United States Sanitary Commission during the Civil War. As a young woman, Aldrich worked with Clara Barton in the Red Cross and operated a field hospital in Puerto Rico for the Army during the Spanish–American War. By 1901, she helped pass the bill creating the Women's Army Nursing Corps (Aldrich, 1958; Armeny, 1983; Sarnecky, 1999). She understood the efforts of early nursing leaders to professionalize nursing and recognized the relevance of the Town and Country Nursing Service and rural health care in her community.

Clement also stressed the importance of a nursing advisory committee to establish a viable nursing service in Red Hook. She recommended that the membership should be "constituted of active and broad-minded women, whose supreme thought is the welfare of the community and how the visiting nurse may meet the broadest needs" (Clement, 1916a, p. 1). Aldrich fit Clement's description of a good board member, as did many others in the community, such as physicians, lawyers, and clergymen (Clement, 1986 [sic], p. 1). The committee met weekly and

(continued)

CASE STUDY: The American Red Cross Town and Country *(continued)*

by November 1916, it formed Red Hook Nursing Association in affiliation with the Town and Country Nursing Service (Clement, 1916b).

By 1916, Red Hook leaders had raised sufficient funds to hire their first Town and Country rural public health nurse, Margaret Ruba. Her work focused on school nursing, and within the first month of her arrival she visited children in the four districts of the town. Out of the 261 children she assessed, she identified health-related problems in 184 children. She observed dental and vision problems, enlarged tonsils, nasal obstruction, and other deformities. In addition, she reported that by December 1916, she had made a total of 131 home visits and had given 16 health-related talks to a variety of schools, organizations, and businesses ("A Large Field for Our Red Cross Nurses' Work," December 8, 1916). Her work included a wide array of public health nursing services, including home visits, school nursing, and health education. She traveled throughout the community, providing these services and referring those in need of additional care to the appropriate settings. Ruba served only 1 year in Red Hook, but the town continued to hire a Town and Country rural public health nurse until the 1930s.

The Town and Country Nursing Service affiliation in Red Hook, New York, illustrates how a community recognized a need to provide access to health care to populations within their rural community. To do so, they developed a nursing advisory committee, whose membership reflected representation from a variety of interested stakeholders; used data found in a county-wide survey about the health needs of the community to justify the need for a public health nurse; established a visiting nurse service in the community affiliating with the Town and Country Nursing Service; and hired a Town and Country rural public health nurse that worked toward improving health care outcomes in the community within her first year of service. This effort exemplifies primary health care where a variety of stakeholders come together to address the health of those living in the community (Lewenson, 2017).

DISCUSSION AND CONCLUSION

Public health nursing—an emerging professional role during the early 20th century—required the additional education that prepared these nurses to serve in rural communities. These nurses integrated the art of nursing with the advances in science that aimed to promote a healthier population. They needed to understand the connection between illness and what we call today the determinants of health, such as poor nutrition and poverty (Healthy People 2020, 2015). They brought care into the communities where people lived, worked, and played. The ideas of health prevention and social justice, considered the "dominant note of modern philanthropy," replaced an earlier notion of "charity and relief" (Dixon, 1913, p. 179). Nursing leaders of the day, such as Lillian Wald and Fannie Clement, sought to bring public health ideals into the community in the early 20th century.

The early public health nurses, especially those in rural settings, needed new skills that afforded them the ability to communicate, educate, and negotiate with other stakeholders in a community. They endured travelling long distances between their patients, isolation from other nursing professionals, and limited social support services typically available in cities. Public health nurses in urban settings were more likely to work in either a visiting nurse–type service that cared for the sick at home, or in a larger health department where their work was more about disease prevention and health education. These divisions of service blended in rural communities, as most often these rural nurses provided the sole source of health care access (Lewenson, 2013; Roberts & Heinrich, 1985).

The role of public health nurses advanced during the early 20th century, and continues to evolve today. Public health nurses fit within a primary health care philosophical approach to health, where access to health care, interprofessional collaboration, and use of evidence-based data to support their work, along with an understanding of the determinants of health, contribute to the multidimensional role of public health nursing. Today's public health nurses must have the knowledge, skills, and understanding to be health care advocates for the public they serve. That means, when reading the newspaper about measles epidemics or physicians' home visits, public health nurses must be able to articulate the role of the public health nurse in those circumstances and how their specialized role contributes to public health. It also means knowing how the past informs this evolving role, reflecting Dock and Stewart's (1931) idea that "no occupation can be intelligently followed or understood unless it is, at least to some extent, illumined by the light of history interpreted from the human stand-point" (p. 3). The public health nurse's role, like all other roles in the profession, would benefit from the knowledge that historical back-ground can lend. Fairman and D'Antonio (2013) explained:

> nurses' success in moving policy forward will depend on their ability to give voice to a historical perspective that rec-ognizes the political and contextual forces that shape health care and places nurses and nursing at the center of long-standing debates about health services delivery, knowledge formation, patient safety, technology, and education for practice. (p. 351)

Knowledge of the American Red Cross Town and Country's foray into rural public health nursing allows us to imagine the meaning of public health nursing within primary health care. Nurses learned to col-laborate, communicate, and negotiate with others both at the national and local levels. They needed to understand what it meant to live in rural settings, away from access to care when dealing with infectious dis-eases, when caring for chronic illness, when providing health teaching to young mothers, or when dealing with accidents and emergencies.

Wald's vision for the public health nurse's role reached far beyond the point of service idea to embrace what today we identify as a holis-tic primary health care framework. She identified the determinants of health both in the city and in rural communities, creating organizations, such as the Town and Country Nursing Service, to address the social and physical environments that affected the health of the populations living within the communities. Nurses such as Ruba who worked in Red Hook provided care to the sick, gave educational talks to various groups, and worked with community activists. She, along with the other educated Town and Country nurses, saw their role as broader than just the care of the sick. If they were committed to Wald's ideas, then their role included a commitment to create healthier commu-nities, whether at the bedside, in the schools, or in the political arena. As contemporary public health nurses work toward creating a culture of health, their role must include collaborating with others in local, national, and global communities, in both the public and private sectors, and seeking strong intersectorial ties to bring about change. The value that the leaders of a small community in rural New York placed on the health and well-being of its citizens and its affiliation with the Town and Country Nursing Service illustrates early 20th-century efforts to promote the goals of Healthy People 2020, which continue to underpin the practice of the public health nurse today.

ACTIVITIES FOR TEACHING AND LEARNING

1. Examine a local newspaper and identify how many stories, references, or editorials are published that address a public health nursing issue? Does the story reflect urban or rural public health concerns? What strategies could a public health nurse (rural or urban) initiate to improve the health of the public in that community?
2. Look at your own community and identify three priority health needs that exist. Then look at the census data for the community that span over a 50-year period. What public health nursing measures would the nurse in the community be able to develop as part of a nurse-run nursing initiative?
3. Explore three different stakeholders in your community who would support a public health nursing initiative. What skills would a public health nurse need to collaborate with these stakeholders?
4. Discuss the rationale for understanding the historical development of the public health nursing role and advocacy for health care policy today.

REFERENCES

A Large Field for Our Red Cross Nurses' Work. (1916, December 8). *Tivoli Times.* Retrieved from http://www.worldcat.org/identities/nc-red%20hook%20 nursing%20association%20red%20hook%20n%20y

Aldrich, M. C. (1916, April 6). Red Cross rural nurses: To the editor of the Tivoli Times. *Tivoli Times.* Retrieved from http://www.worldcat.org/identities/ nc-red%20hook%20nursing%20association%20red%20hook%20n%20y

Aldrich, M. C. (1958). *Family vista: The memoirs of Margaret Chanler Aldrich.* Collections of the Dutchess County Historical Society (Vol. VIII). New York, NY: William-Frederick Press.

American Public Health Association. (2013). The definition and practice of public health nursing: A statement of the APHA public health nursing section.

Retrieved from http://apha.org/~/media/files/pdf/membergroups/nurs ingdefinition.ashx

Armeny, S. (1983). Organized nurses, woman philanthropists and the intellectual bases for cooperation among women, 1898–1920. In E. C. Lagemann (Ed.), *Nursing history: New perspectives, new possibilities* (pp. 13–45). New York, NY: Teachers College Press.

Buhler-Wilkerson, K. (1993). Public health then and now: Bringing care to the people: Lillian Wald's legacy to public health nursing. *American Journal of Public Health, 83*(12), 1778–1782.

Clement, F. F. (1916a, March 18). Letter from Fannie F. Clement to Miss Mary Gerard Lewis. Red Hook Nursing Association Records (Box 362.104 R). Adriance Memorial Library, Poughkeepsie, NY.

Clement, F. F. (1916b, November). The Red Cross. *American Journal of Nursing, 17*(2), 147–149. Retrieved from http://www.jstor.org/stable/3406226

Clement, F. F. (1986 [*sic*], July 26). Letter from Fannie F. Clement to Miss Mary Gerard Lewis. Red Hook Nursing Association Records (Box 362.104 R). Adriance Memorial Library, Poughkeepsie, NY.

DeVille, K., & Novick, L. (2011). Swimming upstream? Patient Protection and Affordable Care Act and the cultural ascendancy of public health. *Journal Public Health Management, 17*(2), 102–109.

Dixon, M. B. (1913, September). Editorials: The domestic educator and the immigrant. *The Johns Hopkins Nurses Alumna Magazine, 12*(3), 178–181.

Dock, L. L., Pickett, S. E., Clement, F. F., Fox, E. G., & Van Meter, A. R. (1922). *History of American Red Cross nursing* (p. 1213). New York, NY: Macmillan.

Dock, L. L., & Stewart, I. M. (1931). *A short history of nursing: From the earliest times to the present day* (3rd ed., text rev.). New York, NY: G. P. Putnam's Sons.

Fairman, J., & D'Antonio, P. (2013). History counts: How history can shape our understanding of health policy. *Nursing Outlook, 61*(5), 346–352.

Greenhalgh, T. (2007). *Primary health care: Theory and practice.* Malden, MA: Blackwell Publishing.

Hassmiller, S. B. (2017). Nursing's role in building a culture of health. In S. B. Lewenson & M. Truglio-Londrigan (Eds.), *Practicing primary health care in nursing: Caring for populations* (pp. 33–60). Sudbury, MA: Jones & Bartlett.

Healthy People 2020. (2015). Determinants of health. Washington, DC: Office of Disease Prevention and Health Promotion. Retrieved from http://www .healthypeople.gov/2020/about/foundation-health-measures/Determina nts-of-Health

Institute of Medicine. (1988). *The future of public health*. Washington, DC: National Academies Press.

Jauhar, S. (2015, October 14). Bring back house calls. *New York Times*, the Opinion Pages, Op–Ed. Retrieved from http://www.nytimes.com/2015/10/15/opinion/bring-back-house-calls.html

Keeling, A., & Lewenson, S. B. (2013). A nursing historical perspective on the medical home: Impact on health care policy. *Nursing Outlook, 61*(5), 360–366. doi:10.1016/j.outlook.2013.07.003

Kernodle, P. B. (1949). *The Red Cross nurse in action: 1882–1948*. New York, NY: Harper & Brothers.

Lewenson, S. B. (1993). *Taking charge: Nursing suffrage, and feminism in America, 1873–1920*. New York, NY: Garland Publishing.

Lewenson, S. B. (2013). Public health nursing in the United States: A history. In M. Truglio-Londrigan & S. B. Lewenson (Eds.), *Public health nursing: Practicing population-based care* (2nd ed., pp. 25–51). Burlington, MA: Jones & Bartlett.

Lewenson, S. B. (2015). Town and Country nursing: Community participation and nurse recruitment. In J. C. Kirchgessner & A. W. Keeling (Eds.), *Nursing rural America: Perspectives from the early 20th century* (pp. 1–19). New York, NY: Springer Publishing.

Lewenson, S. B. (2017). Primary health care: Exemplar from nursing history. In S. B. Lewenson & M. Truglio-Londrigan (Eds.), *Primary health care in nursing: Population-based care* (pp. 21–31). Burlington, MA: Jones & Bartlett.

Lewenson, S. B., & Truglio-Londrigan, M. (2017). Preface. In S. B. Lewenson & M. Truglio-Londrigan (Eds.), *Primary health care in nursing: Population-based care* (pp. xi–xix). Burlington, MA: Jones & Bartlett.

Nightingale, F. (1893/1949). Sick nursing and health nursing: Addendum. District nursing. In I. A. Hampton and others (Eds.), *Nursing of the sick 1893: Papers and discussions from the International Congress of Charities, Correction and Philanthropy, Chicago* (published in 1949 under the sponsorship of the National League of Nursing Education, pp. 24–43). New York, NY: McGraw-Hill.

Roberts, D. E., & Heinrich, J. (1985). Public health nursing comes of age. *American Journal of Public Health, 75*(10), 1162–1172.

Sarnecky, M. T. (1999). *A history of the U.S. Army Nurse Corps*. Philadelphia: University of Pennsylvania Press.

State Charities Aid Association. (1915). *Sickness in Dutchess County, New York: Its extent, care, and prevention* (Book No. 136, pp. 1–119). New York, NY: Author.

Retrieved from https://babel.hathitrust.org/cgi/pt?id=mdp.390150685610 45;view=1up;seq=5

Truglio-Londrigan, M., & Lewenson, S. B. (2013). What is public health and public health nursing? In M. Truglio-Londrigan & S. B. Lewenson (Eds.), *Public health nursing: Practicing population-based care* (2nd ed., pp. 3–23). Burlington, MA: Jones & Bartlett.

Truglio-Londrigan, M., Singleton, J., Lewenson, S. B., & Lopez, L. (2013). Conversation about primary health care. In M. Truglio-Londrigan & S. B. Lewenson (Eds.), *Public health nursing: Practicing population-based care* (2nd ed., pp. 399–411). Burlington, MA: Jones & Bartlett.

Turkewitz, J., & Cave, D. (2015, January 30). As measles cases speak in U.S., so does anxiety. Retrieved from http://www.nytimes.com/2015/01/31/us/as -measles-spreads-in-us-so-does-anxiety.html?_r=

U.S. Department of Health and Human Services. (2010). Healthy People 2020 framework. Retrieved from http://www.healthypeople.gove/20202/about/ default.aspx

Wald, L. D. (1913). Address by the president of the National Organization for Public Health Nurses: Report of the Sixteenth Annual Convention. *American Journal of Nursing, 13*(12), 924–926.

Wald, L. D. (1918a, March 5). *The woman voter should realize the relation of the visiting nurse to public health: The designer.* Lillian Wald Papers (Writings & Speeches, Voters & Voting, Reel 25, p. 1). New York Public Library, New York, NY.

Wald, L. D. (1918b, May). *Address at Graduation Johns Hopkins Hosptial—May 1, 1918.* Lillian Wald Papers (Writings & Speeches, Nurses & Nursing II, Reel 25, pp. 1–12). New York Public Library, New York, NY.

Wald, L. D. (1921, October 6). *Address at the Red Cross Convention, Columbus, Ohio. The Henry Street Nurse, 2*(10–11), 1–4. Lillian Wald Papers (Writings & Speeches, Nurses & Nursing, Reel 25). New York Public Library, New York, NY.

Whelan, J. (2015, October 22). The nurse will see you now (at home). Retrieved from http://historian.nursing.upenn.edu/2015/10/22/the-nurse-will-see -you-now-at-home

Chapter 3: School Nursing: A Challenging Strategy in Rural Health Care in the United States

MARY ECKENRODE GIBSON

The children of today must be viewed as the raw material of a new State; the schools as the nursery of the Nation.

(Hoag & Terman, 1914, p. 4)

Child Health is the corner-stone of the edifice of public health and community welfare. A stream can rise no higher than its source. Childhood is the source of the Nation.

(Keene, 1929, p. 1)

Health and education affect individuals, society and the economy and as such, must work together whenever possible. Schools are a perfect setting for this collaboration.

(ASCD, 2014, p. 3)

These statements, dating from 1914, 1929, and 2014, were written by education professionals. Today's philosophy still reflects the protective and hopeful beliefs of leaders in education of 100 years ago concerning the influence of child health on our nation's future. What happens in our schools has a huge impact on the future of our country; therefore, keeping children in school, healthy and ready to learn, is a universal goal throughout the United States. Yet today, with the student population reflecting more children with disabilities and huge health disparities, we still have no comprehensive national health program in place for our school children. With these past and present views on the importance of child health, why is it that over the past 100 years we have not achieved a coherent and universal plan for healthy school children in our country?

This chapter aims to examine today's demand for school nurses, and to articulate the early 20th-century history of school nursing, particularly in rural areas. By linking the efforts of the past to the goals of today, we hope to allow history to be our "wise teacher," not just teaching us who we are but also outlining a way to understand current issues that can lead us to insights about our future (Lewenson & Herrmann, 2008, pp. 1–2). Public health nurses led school nursing efforts a century ago and their work illustrates some surprising similarities to challenges that we face today. These include inconsistent funding, inadequate numbers of nurses in this role, and the sovereignty of local and state politics.

The National Association of School Nurses (NASN) defines school nursing as "a specialized practice of professional nursing that advances the well-being, academic success and lifelong achievement and health of students" (NASN, 2012, p. 2). The nurse in the school setting facilitates normal development, promotes health and safety, intervenes with health problems, provides case management, collaborates to help students and families adapt and manage, and advocates for students and their learning (Council on School Health, 2008; NASN, 2012). The NASN, founded in 1979, is the professional organization that advances the practice of school nurses, envisioning that every student will thus be healthy, safe, and ready to learn. The NASN definition places the nurse at the center of health management at the school level, partnering with the school system, local physicians, and the public, and argues for the importance of having a school nurse in every school, yet fulltime RNs currently staff only about half of U.S. schools (Robert Wood Johnson Foundation [RWJF], 2010).

A recent publication stresses that "schools are situated within the contexts of neighborhoods and communities. The relationship between the school and the community affects the entire community, not just the students attending the school" (Lewallen, Hunt, Potts-Datema, Zaza, & Giles, 2015, p. 736). School nurses have played a key role in forging healthy communities during the past century. In the early 20th century, just as today, an environment conducive to learning (both inside and outside of the classroom) was key to the health and success of school children, and indeed to communities and our nation. The physical environment of schools, as well as the physical condition of learners, have played huge roles in the strategies to improve school health. Today, a collaborative approach called "Whole School, Whole Community, Whole Child" (ASCD, 2014) currently underpins federal efforts to coordinate learning and health. The aim of this program is to provide holistic school programs to enhance students' ability to learn by promoting healthy students and providing a healthy environment and access to health and behavioral services when needed. In fact, the whole student has been a focus of school nursing since its inception. Schools can be a gateway for some students to needed health services today just as they were in the past.

"Parents have to send their children to schools; they do not have to take them to private physicians' and dentists' offices or to public clinics," argued Meckel (2013, p. 1) in his book, *Classrooms and Clinics: Urban Schools and the Protection and Promotion of Child Health*. Children are required to attend school but not required to access routine medical services. Having a nurse in the school encourages a link between the school and the health care system and promotes preventive care and health education, as well as provides for therapeutic care for some students. Today's school nurses regularly treat or manage asthma, allergies, and chronic diseases such as diabetes; advise and counsel students on behavioral, substance abuse, or sexuality issues and prevention strategies; provide vision and hearing screening and immunization monitoring; and treat minor injuries (RWJF, 2010). The ability of today's school children to be present and ready to learn includes some newer challenges, which affect the scope of practice of the school nurse.

Policy and Political Advocacy

Several key legislative events influenced the scope of school nurses' work. In 1973, the Rehabilitation Act required access to public education for students with disabilities and required individualized services to be in place to accommodate their learning. The Individuals with Disabilities Education Act (IDEA) of 1975 and 1997 mandated that schools admit and provide educational services for children with disabilities, ranging from psychological and developmental services to physical services, sometimes for debilitating and chronic diseases. These two Acts virtually redefined the school population for public education, and required adjustments for even the most disabled children to be accommodated in the classroom in the least restrictive way.

These Acts essentially mandated that nursing services be provided for students, but failed to provide funding for such services (Wolfe & Selekman, 2002).

To provide some perspective on the scope of the issue, a U.S. Census Bureau study indicates that 5% of the children in metropolitan areas and 6.3% in nonmetropolitan areas have a disability (Brault, 2011). This adds up to a total of 2.8 million children with disabilities who need individualized services ranging from blood glucose testing to tracheostomy care (Brault, 2011; Wang et al., 2014). Add to this total the 8% of children (nearly 6 million, or one in 13) with food allergies who can experience life-threatening reactions while in school and more than 9% of children with asthma (approximately 6.8 million), and the acute need for qualified RNs in every school becomes clear (Centers for Disease Control and Prevention [CDC], 2015a; Food Allergy Research and Education [FARE], 2015).

In addition, health disparities affect countless students. The term *health disparity* refers to a higher burden of illness, injury, disability, or mortality experienced by a group of people relative to another group (Kaiser Family Foundation, 2012). For example, impoverished families and persons of color experience worse health outcomes than other populations in the United States—they have poorer access to care, have poorer quality care, and are less likely to be insured. Health disparities contribute substantially to excess health care costs in the United States (Kaiser Family Foundation, 2012). In 2013, more than one in five children lived below the poverty level in the United States (Annie E. Casey Foundation, 2014). Other factors such as environmental threats, individual and behavioral factors, and educational inequalities enhance the disparity issues for school-age children (CDC, 2015b) and further document the need for nurses in schools.

Healthy People 2020 (Educational and Community-Based Programs [ECBP]—Objective 5; 2016) aims to increase the proportion of elementary, middle, and senior high schools that have a full-time school nurse (defined as an RN or a licensed practical nurse [LPN]) to student ratio of at least 1:750. In fact, 45% of the U.S. public schools met this challenge in 2006, and now the goal is to increase the ratio by 10% by 2020 (Healthy People.gov, n.d.). Further recommendations by the Council on School Health (2008) and the American Academy of Pediatrics (AAP) propose that schools with larger numbers of children with special health needs require more intensive nurse-to-student ratios. State laws and guidelines vary tremendously on this issue (see National Association of State Boards of Education [NASBE], 2014). For example, Iowa requires schools and school districts to employ a school nurse (RN) with at least a bachelor's degree, and allows care to be delegated within the school to an LPN (NASBE, 2014). Iowa further set the goal of a nurse-to-student ratio of 1:750. In contrast, Virginia school boards may employ nurses if they meet certain Board of Education criteria, and local health departments may also provide personnel for health services in the school system. The Virginia law stipulates that skilled nursing services paid for by Medicaid must be performed by an RN or LPN under the supervision of an RN. The law recommends one nurse per 1,000 students (NASBE, 2014), but these recommendations are an unfunded mandate.

In light of these statistics, it is astonishing to learn (even after 100 years of advocacy), that not all schools have an RN on site to serve the child and adolescent population as well as provide health promotion and health education in the schools. In fact, there are 73,600 RNs working in schools in the capacity of a school nurse, though not all are full time (Turner, 2016). In many areas of the country, depending on state laws, other paraprofessionals or lay persons may fill the role of a health clinician. These raw data numbers of nurses (73,600) as compared to the public and private school student numbers (50.1 million plus 4.9 million; National Center for Educational Statistics, 2015) might suggest an adequate force of school nurses (1:747); however, that figure disguises wide differences across the country. A recent survey documented that various regions of the country differ significantly in terms of nurse-to-student ratios—some more than double the recommended 1:750 ratio—and in terms of salary paid to nurses (NASN, 2012; Figure 3.1). A "patchwork of state and local policies on nurse practice and standards as well as inconsistent and sometimes fractured systems of financing" creates challenges for school nursing advocates (RWJF, 2010, p. 1).

Multiple professional groups endorse the need for the services of school nurses, such as the AAP, the National Education Association (NEA, 2015), the NASN, the American Nurses Association (ANA), and CDC, to name only a few. The *Journal of the American Medical Association* recently published a report documenting the cost-effectiveness of school nursing and noted that for every dollar invested in school nursing, society would gain $2.20 (Wang et al., 2014). The school nurse focuses

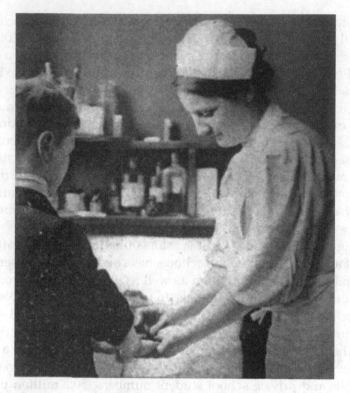

FIGURE 3.1 Mrs. Edith McCarl Hickey.
Source: Sunset Magazine (1915, p. 552).

on education and prevention, but deals with more chronic medical conditions than acute ones. The nurse's role not only saves health care costs, but provides that link to the health care system. A discussion of the past provides some perspective for the present.

BACKGROUND

Children born around the turn of the 20th century in the United States, depending on their location and race, had as high as a one-in-five chance of dying before their fifth birthday (Markel, 1998). Diseases such as measles, diphtheria, smallpox, systemic infections, and tuberculosis (TB), along with regional diseases such as pellagra or parasitic diseases such as malaria and hookworm, threatened children's lives—that is, if they survived infancy. Impure milk and water led to gastroenteritis and diarrhea that along with respiratory infections claimed the lives of countless babies even before their first birthday (Golden, Meckel, & Prescott, 2004). Black children died twice as frequently as White children, and poorer children were subject to greater mortality as well (Brosco, 1999). In fact, the Children's Bureau, founded in 1912, the first federal agency to address children's health and needs, noted in one of its first studies that decreasing income was correlated with increasing infant mortality. The babies of the lowest wage earners and those of single mothers were more than twice as likely to die as those of the highest wage earners (Lathrop, 1919; Lindenmeyer, 1997). Some public health activists called cities children's "abattoirs" (slaughterhouses), but rural children had different, yet equally challenging obstacles to surmount in order to achieve and maintain health, so critical to academic success.

In contrast to the perception of rural good health were challenges such as poverty, poor sanitation, child farm labor, parasitic infections, and skin infections along with infectious diseases and accidents. In addition, school terms lasted as little as 72 days in rural areas, and ramshackle school buildings were hardly optimal places for learning (Flannagan, 1914; Link, 1986). One public health nurse leader stated, "Unless one has actually visited the families living on small isolated farms, it is hard to realize the meaning of the poverty in many rural areas" (Randall, 1931, p. 193). In addition to isolated family or sharecropping farm work, there was mining, forges, wood cutting, saw mills, and other, often low-paying, rural labor pursuits that could bring this type of poverty into focus. A public health nurse in Washington state described her initial work in King County, "I spent one week among the mining camps, and the squalor of the homes, combined with the general neglect of the children, made my heart ache" (Hickey, 1913, p. 166). With poverty often comes poor health.

Public health professionals of the time sought innovative tactics to fight diseases and promote health in these rustic populations, yet school nursing was a consistent choice to address children's health (Meckel, 1990) and was considered by many the most effective way of introducing public health nursing in a rural community (Brainard, 1922/1985). Discussing rural nursing, one author in the *American Journal of Nursing* stated, "In a great many cases the children are the only means of reaching the homes, sometimes situated in such out-of-the-way places that it is hard to find them" (Koeller, 1917, p. 317). Schools not only needed the services of the nurse, but also supplied the access to the children's families in these often remote regions. It is hard for us today to imagine the unpaved, rutted roads, or mere pathways over rough terrain that led to rural homes. These factors dictated the means of travel for those who visited. Although these issues may sound far different from our current experience, we have much to learn from the strategies that our nursing and public health counterparts used 100 years ago.

Origin of School Nursing

In 1892, Nurse Amy Hughes went into several London elementary schools located in poor neighborhoods. She examined up to 100 children a day—referred by teachers—and treated simple, contagious infections such as ringworm and pediculosis (lice) without excluding children from schools, thus keeping children in the classroom and ready to learn (Brainard, 1922/1985). The successes of Amy Hughes and a growing contingent of school nurses around London at the turn of the century suggested that the nurse, "for small ills, might be more useful than the doctor—identifying and treating head lice, eye disease, promoting cleanliness and referring the children to medical care if needed" (Report of the Commissioner of Education, 1906, p. 163). In 1897, London's programs were recognized in New York City, where, using a different tactic, doctors began to inspect children in the city schools.

Physician medical inspectors excluded children who needed treatment from school, and sent them home with notices recommending parents seek treatment for the child. Parents often ignored or did not respond to the notice. Absences persisted and the goal of keeping children in the classroom to learn was not met, and children often remained an exposure risk in their families or neighborhoods.

School Nursing in New York City

Public health nursing leader Lillian Wald, fully aware of the work in London, offered the city schools the loan of a Henry Street Settlement nurse, Lina Rogers, to supplement the work of the inspecting doctors. Rogers visited four schools in a densely populated area of the city and followed up the inspections with in-school treatment when possible and paid home visits to the families of the children to ensure that appropriate management of the problem and health education occurred. Many of the exclusions involved skin diseases (such as ringworm, scabies, impetigo), which, when "treated" on site at the school with soap, water, and ointments, or simple remedies, allowed the children to return to school. Rogers also documented and treated cases of pediculosis, eczema, eye infections, and minor wounds (Keeling, 2007). This month-long experiment in the fall of 1902 proved so successful that the city ultimately employed 12 nurses by the end of that year, and Lina Rogers became the superintendent of the work.

During the first year of school nurses in New York City schools, the monthly absentee rate dropped from 10,500 to 1,100 (Rogers, 1908). Rogers declared, "The care given to the children in the schools is the ameliorative, that given in the homes is the preventive part of the whole." She considered home visits to be "by far the most important" (Rogers, 1906, p. 67). Another physician advocate later declared, " . . . it is impracticable to disassociate the school nurse from the home in successful school work" (Clark, 1922, p. 2193). These school nurses focused primarily on acute health issues. Urban schools began to adopt school nursing across the continent as programs launched in Chicago, Los Angeles, Boston, Pueblo, Colorado, and Toronto, Canada, within the first 10 years, and Rogers went on to become a leader in school nursing. But at the turn of the 20th century, only 40% of the population resided in urban environments (Iowa Data Center, n.d.; U.S. Census, n.d.).

Rural School Nursing

Rural schools, serving the other 60% of the population, faced many of the same health and social issues as urban ones. Many of these children were also poor, yet they had the additional burdens of isolation, dilapidated school houses, lack of public and private sanitation, and inadequate access to health care resources, along with unique social challenges. Throughout the country, such diseases as typhoid and TB, infected ears, trachoma, dysentery, malnutrition, and poor vision hampered rural children's learning. In the South, malaria and hookworm were added to the list. Conditions in the schools promoted the spread of many of these infections. In the 1910s, multiple educational sources documented the lack of sanitary privies, clean water, and schoolhouse conditions that obstructed learning (Clark, 1914; Flannagan, 1914). Further environmental issues, now viewed as social determinants of health, also existed. As one social welfare worker put it, "Poverty and neglect, vice and crime, disease and death do not pertain exclusively to cities, nor do laziness and ignorance" (Curry, 1923, p. 200). Experts noted irregular school attendance, poor nutrition, lack of good employ-ment for parents, and inadequate housing in these rural areas.

One cannot consider the early 20th-century proposed reforms in public education, including healthy conditions for learning and the role of the school in society, without considering the ambiguity of pro-gressive reform for the rural population. This ambiguity lies in the understanding of two conflicting ideologies—the concurrent drive to modernize and use science to reform societal problems, and the proud demand to preserve the independent, entrenched values of the provin-cial way of life. Modernization, or progressivism, therefore could con-ceivably unravel the traditional way of life, so dear to country people (Link, 1983). One school nursing proponent observed that "to awaken these good rural parents from their conservatism and to the necessity of safeguarding the physical welfare of their children" is one of the most important missions of the rural nurse (Cannon, 1921, p. 132).

Another noted (Stebbins, 1929):

> . . . we find our rural Missouri communities large in area, often handicapped by meager transportation . . . financially struggling . . . with an unawakened group consciousness, barely stirring . . . a surrounding open country peopled with . . . individualistically thinking and acting, self-reliant agriculturalists; a divergence of thinking between the town and open-country people; and in . . . sections of the state special racial and industrial problems. (p. 27)

School nursing in rural areas was a connecting link between the emerg-ing bureaucratic systems of education and public health.

In the South, one public health nursing leader stated that although training was important, it was equally important "that we have south-ern women to do the work, as they understand conditions so much bet-ter than do nurses coming from the more prosperous North" (Virginia State Board of Health and State Health Commissioner, 1916, p. 138). This supports the notion that the rural nurse faced a double-edged role: as a reformer and improver of rural health and sanitation while treading a fine line to preserve rural identity; change was not easily accepted. Leaders recognized that having nurses come from the region where they would work had value and might not tip that bal-ance that could derail the modernization efforts if rural values were not sustained.

School nurses, as representatives of their profession at the time, became the "entering wedge" to rural communities and schools, with the confidence that "the teaching of the nurse will be carried home through the child" (Ludwig, 1916, p. 76). Localities and schools first had to recognize that they needed this service, since funding was mostly local, and then they needed to locate a nurse who could meet the demanding criteria. Frequently hired by school boards but also funded through piecemeal sources, such as mothers' clubs, local funds, parent teacher associations (PTAs), the Red Cross, and later by state health departments, school nurses tackled school children's health and sanitation problems head on. They identified individual health problems in the schools, visited homes to seek consent for care, assessed whole families and their environments, and followed up with medical and nursing care (Figure 3.2). Whether or not the nurse had a medical inspector to assist in the work was a local decision. Physician inspectors were expensive, and had their own medical practices to tend. Authorities agreed that if the funds were available for only one health officer in a small town, the nurse was the most effective choice (Cabot, 1911).

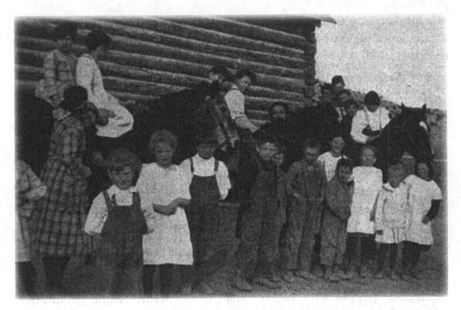

FIGURE 3.2 Waiting for the nurse.
Source: Wiberg (1921, p. 167).

Certainly, there were challenges for the nurse—not only in funding but also rural transportation, physical isolation, sheer distance between schools, living quarters, and social and professional isolation. For example, one Missouri nurse opined:

> Roads, their direction and condition, are a definite determining factor. It is sometimes necessary . . . to go many more miles . . . just because there is no road to the nearest . . . village, or its upkeep is so inferior . . . [for] it to be used. Sometimes, too, the "creeks are up." (Stebbins, 1929, p. 25)

The nurse could face parental indifference and lack of understanding of the need for the nurse's health message. In addition, there were often few available hospitals and clinics where parents could take their children for care. Nurses had to face pushback from the medical profession at times if they advocated for free or reduced cost care (Johnson, 1936; Kelly, 1921; Waterman, 1934; Williamson, 1927). In order to do their work, nurses were obliged to navigate and partner with local officials, school officials, teachers, physicians, the community, and the students and parents under their care, who often represented diverse interests and priorities.

The scope of the job itself remained a consistent barrier to adequate school nursing. Nurses might be hired to do school work, but as one teacher noted:

> Her opportunity for service is limited only by her strength, her endurance and her vision. In many cases she is the leader in welfare activities of the community and takes the initiative not only in developing the school health program, but in organizing . . . the improvement of the health of school children. (Williamson, 1927, p. 392)

Rima Apple (2015), historian of public health nursing, contended that local funding and a supportive infrastructure influenced public health developments, including school nursing. "It was difficult for a single person, even a highly competent person, to sustain a job 'so large,' with 'so much to accomplish,' and at the same time ill-defined and so easily expanded" (Apple, 2015, p. 35). This infrastructure would eventually take the form of local health units that could support the work of the nurse, but was long in coming to many rural areas of the United States.

Historical Attributes of a Rural School Nurse

To be successful, the rural nurse needed to possess an almost impossible list of attributes. Of all qualities, tact and a cool head are most frequently cited in the literature (Koeller, 1917). But the nurse also required self-reliance, a 2-year nursing program; a postgraduate course in public health, registration in those states that required it, good health, courage, an even temperament, a sense of humor, a discreet and silent tongue, sympathy with country people, the broadest intelligence, and finally experience in managing a horse [cart] and automobile (Bigbee & Crowder, 1985; Lowe, 1916). One Kentucky nurse advised, "One needs to go into a small town with an open mind, open eyes and ears, but a closed mouth on local conditions regarding her work; but open and well prepared on the work she is going to do" (Lowe, 1916, p. 1187). A successful school nurse required courage, creativity, strong assessment skills, outstanding communication skills, discretion (what we might call emotional intelligence today), and a sense of caring and respect for the community.

> **CASE STUDY: The Case for School Nursing in the 1910s in Virginia**
>
> Virginia State Commissioner of Health, Ennion Williams, demonstrated his favor for school nursing in 1916:
>
> > It is our belief that the school is the first place for the nurse to begin her work . . . by operating in the schools, she can reach a considerable element of the population in a very short while. More than this, the school offers . . . the most effective point of contact between sanitation and the home. The nurse who comes to plead for the treatment of a child is accorded a welcome which a regular health inspector or health officer cannot hope to receive. (Virginia State Board of Health and State Health Commissioner, 1916, p. 69)
>
> Progressive public health officials such as Williams, from primarily rural states, devised ways to intervene with the rural

(continued)

CASE STUDY: The Case for School Nursing in the 1910s
in Virginia *(continued)*

population of the state and saw this challenge as no less than a crusade to improve health and sanitation. Jane Ranson, the first director of Bureau of Public Health Nursing for the state of Virginia, also favored school nursing as the best way to begin or extend work in rural areas, stating, "In country districts school nursing is advocated as having the greatest value, and bringing in the biggest return for the money expended" (Virginia State Board of Health and State Health Commissioner, 1917, p. 169). Schools were a likely place to start and school nursing was a broad yet spotty effort to address those same rural needs—broad in the sense that the nurse could serve multiple roles, and spotty in the sense that there were few nurses available and trained to take on this role that combined nursing, sanitary instruction, and social welfare. Virginia and other states prioritized child health.

Much like urban school nursing began in New York City at the turn of the century, rural school work included direct care, education (for students and teachers), and prevention at the school and during home visits. Inspection led to identification of "defects," as they were called, in vision, hearing, teeth, weight, tonsils, or adenoids. The nurse would treat simple cases according to standing orders and follow up with parents on health issues requiring physician or dentist interventions, such as enlarged or infected tonsils or decayed teeth. Recall that in this preantibiotic era, frequent tonsillitis would have been treated by tonsillectomy; thus, a nurse would have to advocate for a visit to the physician who would schedule the surgery. In fact, in some cases, the nurse organized mass tonsillectomy or dental clinics. For example, Sarah Crosley, RN, organized and set up a makeshift operating room in an Accomack County high school in 1923, where 27 children had their tonsils and adenoids removed by a specialist. They were supported by local doctors, neighboring county nurses, and local volunteers in the care of the children ("With the nurses," 1923, pp. 10–11). Due to

(continued)

CASE STUDY: The Case for School Nursing in the 1910s in Virginia *(continued)*

the scarcity of nurses and physicians in rural areas, along with travel challenges, the rural work demanded initiative, independent judgment, coordination efforts, and a great deal of what one nurse called "cheerful cooperation" (Figure 3.3; Gibbes, 1920, p. 927).

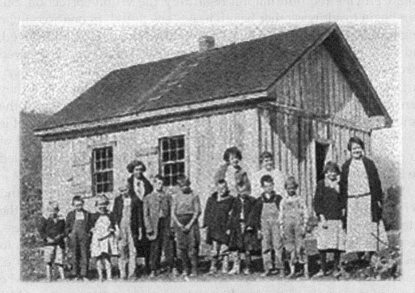

FIGURE 3.3 A typical mountain school.
Source: Ballou (1925, p. 339).

DISCUSSION AND CONCLUSION

School nurses were in the forefront of health promotion and education. In the schools, they taught students healthy patterns of living, such as tooth brushing and healthy eating. Nurses taught children how to drink more milk and to use a handkerchief to cover coughs, and used stories, songs, and poems to cement health messages that they intended for children to share at home. This brand of nursing led to maternal and infant care in the homes visited; discovery of diseases such as TB in families; promotion of sanitation (clean water and sewage disposal); discovery and correction of hookworm, all the while advocating for the correction of vision, nutritional problems, tonsillitis, or the repair of decayed teeth in the school child. For example, a nurse might home visit to investigate a case of a school child's poor vision, with the intent for the parents to take the child to get glasses, but come across a pregnant mother with other small children whose needs she would assess. Perhaps there would be feeding problems or lack of prenatal care. She would provide the information regarding the vision correction, but then begin to address other health issues she found. In one account, a neighbor alerted one nurse to visit a farm where five children lived, and the family's cows appeared sickly. She visited, found, and observed the cows. They were thin and suspicious, so she called the state veterinarian, who visited and found the cows to be tuberculous, and they were euthanized. This nurse's visit likely averted TB infection in the family (Carruthers, 1921). Another expert noted, "The rural school is the way to the improvement of the health of county children and of rural life" (Cannon, 1921). Disease prevention and health promotion led the list of nurse duties.

School nursing could be entirely centered on school children and their families, or it could be only a part of a county nurse's work. In the latter, schools could only occupy part of the nurse's time. Nevertheless, the number of nurses pursuing school nursing was never enough to meet all the needs. The dependence on local funding, the scarcity of qualified nurses for this work, and the thousands of square miles to be covered led many localities to ultimately hire generalist county public health nurses, who could include schools in their work.

The role was incredibly broad and challenging. An example of the work of a school nurse in 1927 provides some perspective:

> I recall one day spent with a rural school nurse who visited seven schools by travelling sixty miles through beautiful mountainous country. As we drove from school to school . . . the nurse [assisted] the teacher in making an annual physical inspection which included the testing of vision and hearing, inspection of teeth and tonsils, and the weighting and measuring of the children. (Williamson, 1927, p. 392)

Another nurse gave an account of her work in rural Utah, "At Strawberry [School] I visited each of the two rooms, gave health talks and made class room inspections, also a thorough inspection of the building, grounds and out-houses, and made recommendations for beautifying and improving the premises" (Wiberg, 1921, p. 168). Following these school activities, home visits would ensue to inform parents of children needing treatment.

Depending on the distances, terrain, and the number of schools that the nurse covered, these inspections might occur only once a year, especially considering the follow-up needed for the children needing further care. One supervising nurse observed, "the nurse . . . each day, in bad weather and good, takes the trail and finds the people; for truly it is not easy to reach schools through the mountains, on roads impassable by automobile or buggy many months in the year and which can only be reached by horseback" (Webb, 1920, p. 840).

From West Virginia to Arkansas, to Mississippi, Utah, Oregon, Virginia, and New York—across the country—the stories of nurses' work, courage, and resourcefulness are recorded in the journals of the era. To be successful, these nurses needed exceptional training and talent. Whether they were navigating muddy or steep roads, conducting toothbrush drills, treating lice with kerosene, locating a crippled child, transporting families to care, carrying specimens to the state lab for hookworm testing, or planning a clinic, these autonomous nurses adopted a broad definition of holistic health that included the environment, socioeconomic status, and sanitary schools and embraced scientific solutions to many rural problems. Organized public health services reached some areas sooner than others, but rural school children still faced health challenges.

Many of the same challenges that school nurses of 100 years ago faced remain today. Children face poverty, health disparities, and environmental challenges in the schools today just as they did 100 years ago. Funding remains a barrier to the provision of school nursing as do appropriate educational preparation, continuing education, and enough qualified nurses to do the work. Some are still not convinced that school nursing is essential, believing that the school secretary can handle most issues. School nurses need to partner with schools to conduct outcome research that will document their effectiveness. Clear associations between school nursing, student readiness for learning, and performance will strengthen the case for more standardized placement of well-qualified RNs in all schools. Finally, all politics are local. Due to the relative autonomy of states in administering educational programs, nurses and schools need to convince local legislators (with data) that school nursing is a good investment.

ACTIVITIES FOR TEACHING AND LEARNING

1. In your community, explore the number of schools, the number of students in those schools, and the number of school nurses in those schools. Identify two main health issues that school nurses experience in those schools. Explore how the school nurse advocates for better health care in local and national legislative policy arenas.
2. Compare and contrast the role of the rural school nurse in the early 20th century with that of the rural school nurse today. Describe the challenges that the school nurse might face in both time periods, noting the similarities and differences.

REFERENCES

Annie E. Casey Foundation. (2014). Thirty-five largest U.S. cities saw increase in child poverty rate between 2005 and 2013. Retrieved from http://datacenter.kidscount.org/data#USA/1/16/17,18,19,20,22,21,2720

Apple, R. (2015). Public nursing rural Wisconsin. In J. C. Kirchgessner & A. W. Keeling (Eds.), *Nursing rural America: Perspectives from the early 20th century* (pp. 21–38). New York, NY: Springer Publishing.

ASCD (formerly known as the Association for Supervision and Curriculum Development). (2014). Whole school, whole community, whole child: A collaborative approach to learning and health. Retrieved from http://www.cdc.gov/healthyschools/wscc/index.htm

Ballou, N. T. (1925). Evolution of rural clinics in Virginia. *Journal of the American Dental Association, 12*(3), 3.

Bigbee, J., & Crowder, E. (1985). The Red Cross rural nursing service: An innovative model of public health nursing delivery. *Public Health Nursing, 2*(2), 109–121.

Brainard, A. (1922/1985). *The evolution of public health nursing.* Philadelphia, PA: W. B. Saunders.

Brault, M. (2011). School-aged children with disabilities in U.S. metropolitan statistical areas. American Community Survey Briefs. U.S Census Bureau. Retrieved from https://www.census.gov/prod/2011pubs/acsbr10-12.pdf

Brosco, J. (1999). The early history of the infant mortality rate in America: A reflection upon the past and a prophesy of the future. *Pediatrics, 103*(2), 478–485.

Cabot, A. (1911). School inspection in small towns. *Boston Medical and Surgical Journal, 164,* 633–634.

Cannon, E. (1921). The field of rural nursing. *The Public Health Nurse, 13*(3), 129–134.

Carruthers, I. E. (1921). A new venture for county nurse. *The Public Health Nurse, 13*(12), 63.

Centers for Disease Control and Prevention. (2015a). Asthma. Retrieved from http://www.cdc.gov/nchs/fastats/asthma.htm

Centers for Disease Control and Prevention. (2015b). Adolescent and school health: Health disparities. Retrieved from http://www.cdc.gov/healthy youth/disparities/index.htm

Clark, T. (1914). The hygiene of rural schools. *Public Health Reports, 37,* 2364–2367.

Clark, T. (1922). The school nurse: Her duties and responsibilities. *Public Health Report, 37*(36), 2193–2205.

Council on School Health. (2008). Policy statement: Role of the school nurse in providing school health services. *Pediatrics, 121*(5), 1052–1056. doi:10.1542/peds.2008-0382

Curry, H. I. (1923). Child welfare in the rural field. *The Annals of the American Academy of Political and Social Science, 105,* 199–205.

Flannagan, R. (1914). Sanitary survey of the schools of Orange County, VA. *United States Bureau of Education Bulletin, 17*(Whole number 590), 1–38.

Food Allergy Research and Education. (2015). Facts and statistics. Retrieved from https://www.foodallergy.org/document.doc?id=194 and https://www.foodallergy.org/facts-and-stats

Gibbes, V. (1920). Establishing good relations. *The Public Health Nurse, 12*(11), 927–930.

Golden, J., Meckel, R., & Prescott, H. (2004). *Children and youth in sickness and in health.* Westport, CT: Greenwood Press.

Healthy People 2020. (2016). ECBP-5.4: Increase the proportion of elementary schools that have a full-time registered school nurse-to-student-ration of at least 1:750. Retrieved from https://www.healthypeople.gov/node/3496/data-details

Hickey, E. M. (1913). Experiences of a rural school nurse. *Trained Nurse and Hospital Review, 9,* 166–168.

Hoag, E., & Terman, L. (1914). *Health work in the schools.* Boston, MA: Houghton Mifflin.

Iowa Data Center. (n.d.). Urban and rural population for the U.S. and all states: 1900–2000. Retrieved from http://www.iowadatacenter.org/datatables/UnitedStates/urusstpop19002000.pdf

Johnson, M. (1936). Rural public health nursing in Minnesota. *Public Health Nursing, 28,* 681–684.

Kaiser Family Foundation. (2012). *Focus on health care disparities: Key facts.* Menlo Park, CA: Author. Retrieved from https://kaiserfamilyfoundation.files.wordpress.com/2012/11/8396-disparities-in-health-and-health-care-five-key-questions-and-answers.pdf

Keeling, A. W. (2007). *Nursing and the privilege of prescription, 1893–2000.* Columbus: The Ohio State Press.

Keene, C. (1929). *The physical welfare of the school child.* Boston, MA: Houghton Mifflin.

Kelly, H. (1921). Some observations on rural work. *Public Health Nursing, 13*(1), 18–20.

Koeller, S. (1917). Rural district nursing. *American Journal of Nursing, 19*(4), 317–319.

Lathrop, J. (1919). Income and infant mortality. *American Journal of Public Health, 9*(4), 270–274.

Lewallen, T., Hunt, H., Potts-Datema, W., Zaza, S., & Giles, W. (2015). The whole school, whole community, whole child model: A new approach for improving educational attainment and healthy development for students. *Journal of School Health, 85*(11), 729–739.

Lewenson, S., & Herrmann, E. (Eds.). (2008). *Capturing nursing history: A guide to historical methods in research.* New York, NY: Springer Publishing.

Link, W. A. (1983). Making the inarticulate speak: A reassessment of public education in the rural south 1870–1920. *Journal of Thought, 18,* 63–75.

Link, W. A. (1986). *A hard country and a lonely road.* Chapel Hill: University of North Carolina Press.

Lowe, A. (1916). Some suggestions for school nursing in a small town. *American Journal of Nursing, 16*(12), 1187–1192.

Ludwig, C. (1916). The county nurse and the country school. *Public Health Nurse Quarterly, 8*, 73–76.

Mangena, A. S., & Maughan, E. (2015). The 2015 NASN school nurse survey. *National Association of School Nurses, 30*(6), 328–335.

Markel, H. (1998). Caring for the foreign born. *Archives of Pediatric and Adolescent Medicine, 152*, 1020–1026.

Meckel, R. (1990). *Save the babies*. Ann Arbor, MI: University of Michigan Press.

Meckel, R. A. (2013). *Classrooms and clinics: Urban schools and the protection and promotion of child health*. New Brunswick, NJ: Rutgers University Press.

National Association of School Nurses. (2012). NASN position statement: Role of the school nurse. Retrieved from http://nas.sagepub.com.proxy.its.vir ginia.edu/content/27/2/103.full.pdf

National Association of State Boards of Education. (2014). State school health policy database. Retrieved from http://www.nasbe.org/healthy_schools/ hs/map.php

National Center for Educational Statistics. (2015). Fast facts: Back to school statistics. Retrieved from http://nces.ed.gov/fastfacts/display.asp?id=372

National Education Association. (2015). A national look at the school nurse shortage. Retrieved from http://www.nea.org/home/35691.htm

Randall, M. G. (1931). Public health nursing service in rural families. *Milbank Memorial Fund Quarterly Bulletin, 9*(4), 189–203.

Report of the Commissioner of Education 1 (Whole number 314). (1906). Washington, DC: Government Printing Office, 163–168.

Robert Wood Johnson Foundation. (2010). School nurses: Keeping children health and ready to learn. Retrieved from http://www.rwjf.org/en/libr ary/articles-and-news/2010/08/school-nurses-keeping-children-healthy -and-ready-to-learn.html

Rogers, L. (1906). Nurses in the public schools of New York City. *Charities and the Commons, 16*, 65–69.

Rogers, L. (1908). Some phases of school nursing. *American Journal of Nursing, 6*(12), 966–974.

Stebbins, M. E. (1929). Nursing in a rural community in Missouri. *American Journal of Nursing, 29*(1), 23–27.

Sunset Magazine. (1915, September). *35*(3), 52.

Turner, L. (2016). The nurse in the schools. In M. Stanhope & J. Lancaster (Eds.), *Public health nursing: Population-centered health care in the community* (9th ed., p. 915). St. Louis, MO: Elsevier.

U.S. Census. (n.d.). U.S. Census 1790–1990. Retrieved from https://www.census .gov/population/censusdata/table-4.pdf

Virginia State Board of Health and State Health Commissioner. (1916). *Annual report of the State Board of Health and the State Health Commissioner to the Governor of Virginia.* Richmond, VA: Davis Bottom.

Virginia State Board of Health and State Health Commissioner. (1917). *Annual report of the State Board of Health and the State Health Commissioner to the Governor of Virginia.* Richmond, VA: Davis Bottom.

Wang, L. Y., Vernon-Smiley, M., Gapinski, M. A., Desisto, M., Maughan, E., & Sheetz, A. (2014). Cost-benefit study of school nursing services. *Journal of the American Medical Association Pediatrics, 168*(7), 642–648. doi:10.1001/ jamapediatrics.2013.544

Waterman, T. (1934). Pioneering in health in the rural schools. *Public Health Nursing, 26,* 29–33.

Webb, B. (1920). Roaming through Virginia with the public health nurse. *The Public Health Nurse, 12*(10), 839–842.

Wiberg, A. (1921). Does it pay to work in the country? *The Public Health Nurse, 13*(4), 167–169.

Williamson, P. (1927). The rural school nurse. *Trained Nurse and Hospital Review, 79,* 392–396.

With the nurses. (1923, July–August). *Virginia Health Bulletin, 15*(Extra no. 10), 10–11.

Wolfe, L. C., & Selekman, J. (2002). School nurses: What it was and what it is. *Pediatric Nursing, 28*(4), 403–407.

Section II: The World at War

Chapter 4: Wartime Nursing: Feeding as Forgotten Practice

JANE BROOKS

Colonel Griffiths of 89 IGH [Indian General Hospital] alerted HQ Burma Command and demanded trained nursing sisters be sent down at once not only to relieve the pressure on the doctors, but to take over the nursing and supervising of these sick men . . . the daily food ration was in short supply, and as for Red Cross comforts there were none. Eventually we went off and found the quarter-master to find out why there were such food shortages and why no Red Cross beverages had been requisitioned for these very sick men. He did not know as he had had no previous experience in such critical situations as these. Despite the absence of specific drugs, it was not many days after our arrival, that with extra beverages and special tit-bits flown in from Calcutta by the RAF [Royal Air Force] the general condition and mood of the patients improved.

(Salter, n.d., p. 124)

This chapter considers the work of British nursing sisters in the challenging world of World War II. During that conflict, British and other Allied nurses worked in all war zones, sometimes under fire, caring for both combatants and civilian patients. The sisters of the Queen Alexandra's Imperial Military Nursing Service (QAIMNS), their Reservists, and the Territorial Army Nursing Service, amalgamated for the duration of the war under the auspices of the QAIMNS (or the QAs, as they are often known), were frequently the only British military female personnel allowed near the frontline. Despite acquiescence to their presence, the place of female nurses in war zones remained contested. The military nurses needed to negotiate the sensitive gender issues of being in a highly masculine space (Dixon Vuic, 2010, loc 176), acting as morale boosters for the troops, all the while working as clinically expert professionals and officers in the British Army.

As a profession, nursing "inhabits the borderlands between the delivery of scientific solutions and the creation of conditions, in patients and their environments that will permit healing" (Brooks & Hallett, 2015, p. 1). As the quote at the beginning of this chapter suggests, one of the most challenging areas of nursing practice in war, a role that encompasses both nurses' understanding of the science of healing and also the conditions created to support the patient's recovery, is the provision of adequate nutrition. The importance of patient feeding to any narrative of war nursing lies in the vital role that it holds in patients' recovery and also the autonomy of practice that nurses experience when caring for patients' nutritional input. Yet this is an overlooked aspect of nursing practice during war. This chapter explores the dilemmas that face nurses in war situations, and the ways in which nurses in the past have challenged the perceptions of the role of trained nurses in wartime.

BACKGROUND

Brooks and Hallett (2015) argue elsewhere that nursing is an essentially humanitarian service, the design and actions of which are directed at the preservation of and support for life. In this understanding, nursing engagement in war appears contradictory, as the purpose of war is to maim and kill (Starns, 2000, p. xii). Nurses in war provide skilled care, but if that care is successful, it is likely that their patients are returned to the frontline, where they may die (D'Antonio, 2002). Indeed, as Griffiths and Jasper (2007) maintain, "war is an antithesis of health on all levels" (p. 92). Yet, when nurses join the military and take on its uniforms, ranks, and military training, they become as much a part of that world as they do of the nursing world, especially in any subsequent deployment to a war zone. The need for an understanding of the duality of the nurse's role and how individual nurses and the profession as a whole manage that duality is required to be considered (Griffiths & Jasper, 2007).

In war, the contested position of female nurses is further exacerbated by cultural expectations of nurses as professionals dedicated to healing and women's place in the hazardous locations of a war zone (Brooks & Hallett, 2015). When the nurse at war is needed to care for the civilian population or the enemy, such dualities can be tested even further as military nurses treat those very people who are seen to have caused injury to their combatant colleagues (Elliot, 2015). Thus, the nurse in war is challenged to be both a nurse and a soldier and to extend civilian nurses' understanding of compassion to include caring for people in highly dangerous environments, where their own lives may be at risk (Finnegan et al., 2016). Nevertheless, Enloe (1988) argues, "nurses serve in combat regardless of official prohibitions. They serve in combat not because of unusual individual bravery, but because they are part of a military structure that needs their *skills* near combat" (p. 106).

In *Fighting Fit: Health, Medicine and War in the Twentieth Century*, Brown (2008) maintains that although the purpose of medicine and the purpose of war appear to be in opposition, "these aims are not totally incompatible"; in order to continue fighting a nation "needs to have the means of repairing the ravages inflicted by war on the human body in order to return its servicemen to action as quickly as possible" (loc 8). The work of the nurse in the support for a dignified death, the provision of physical and emotional comfort, and, what Henderson (1969) called the "performance of those activities contributing to health or its recovery" (p. 4), are all aspects of care that can repair the ravages of war and are thus essential for a war effort. D'Antonio (2002) acknowledges this when she argues that nursing combines both "caring femininity" (p. 7) and clinical expertise and organizational skills. All of these skills and characteristics were brought to the fore by nurses in the care of both combatants and civilians in war zones in World War II and can be exemplified in the range of innovative practices and improvisations that nurses of all Allied nations and in all war zones brought to their wartime work. Nurses took a wide variety of skills to overseas service. These included traditional nursing skills of comfort and hygiene care, technical skills of wound care and medication administration, and some more bizarre skills, such as the carpentry skills required of the American nurses on active service in Iceland (Sarnecky, 1999, p. 180) and gardening skills of both the Canadian and British nurses to support the occupational therapy of their combatant patients with psychological problems (Toman, 2007, p. 152).

Focusing on the involvement of nurses in World War II, this chapter demonstrates the vital importance of RNs and their nursing work on the health, well-being, and recovery of their military and civilian patients. As the nurses in World War II grew in confidence and the

exigencies of war demanded that they take on more scientific technical work, they engaged in the diagnosis, prescription of medications,
and provision of new technologies, such as the administration of peni-
cillin and psychological therapies. However, throughout the war they
also provided traditional aspects of nursing care, such as hygiene,
pain relief, wound care, and the provision of nutrition—work that
they continued to consider of great value in the healing and recovery
of their patients. In order to demonstrate the expertise and innovative
practices that these traditional nursing roles demanded in a war zone,
this chapter examines the critical role that nurses played in the provision of adequate nutrition.

Feeding is considered an essentially feminine role, associated with
domesticity and the family, yet its importance to patient healing was
part of the lexicon of nursing "knowledge" from the earliest years of
nursing reform in the latter half of the 19th century. In *Notes on Nursing:
What It Is and What It Is Not,* Nightingale (1969) informed her reader of
the importance for the nurse "to have a rule of thought about your
patient's diet" (p. 68). In her *A Text-Book of Nursing: For the Use of Training
Schools, Families and Private Students* written in 1902, American nurse
Clara Weeks-Shaw maintained that providing "food for the sick which
will at once be suitable and acceptable is a matter that requires care,
judgment, and ingenuity" (Weeks-Shaw, 1902, p. 178). In war, feeding
work takes on new meanings as civilians caught up in the fighting die
from starvation and fighting men are too weak to return to the frontline. This chapter, therefore, demonstrates how nurses faced the challenges of providing adequate nutrition to heal and provide sustenance
when the access to nutritious food was limited and their patients were
often too weak to eat.

Patient Feeding Work in War

The dietary needs of patients have not been a feature of wartime-
focused medical and nursing texts until quite recently. In *Medicine and
Victory: British Military Medicine in the Second World War,* Harrison (2004)
does consider the appalling diets that caused debility and deficiency
diseases; however, there is no discussion of the work to improve combatant patients' nutrition. Historians of nursing have started to contribute significantly to this crucial yet neglected study over the past few
years, as they have become more interested in the fundamental aspects
of nursing work and the criticality of this work in the medical response

to war. Helmstadter (2015) argues that the work of the nurses in the Crimea was not only about domestic tasks, but in actuality involved complex clinical decision making and skilled nursing work as well. When Helmstadter (2015) acknowledges the importance of feeding patients, she sees it as part of the complexity of nursing work rather than simple basic food preparation. Part of this is related to the difficulties the nurses had in finding nutritious food and ensuring that the soldiers who needed it received it in sufficient quantities to support their health. Dale (2015), with reference to the Second Anglo-Boer War (1899–1902), demonstrates the vital importance of what Meehan (2003) describes as "careful nursing," that is, the provision of "food, fluids and palliatives" (p. 100), in order to support troops' recovery from the main killer, typhoid.

The expansion of histories of nursing in World War I has significantly increased the interest and awareness of the critical place of nurses as those who provide essential care, including the provision of nutritious food. Hallett (2009) argues that "One of the principles nurses were taught was the importance of allowing the wounded or diseased body to heal itself" (p. 107). Although the work of feeding was considered nontechnical and therefore it was usually the orderlies who fed the patients, the nursing sisters supervised the practice because they recognized that "feeding was a necessary prerequisite to the healing process" (Hallett, 2009, p. 107). More recently, Hallett (2014) identifies that, in World War I, many nurses themselves became ill because of inadequate food. If the lack of sustenance caused debility among the otherwise healthy nursing staff, it is understandable that they would fear the effects of poor nutrition on their patients who were injured, diseased, and already malnourished. The realization of the critical importance of sufficient levels of nutritious food to support the healing and recovery of soldiers was such that it led to the appointment of six nurse specialists as dieticians in 1918. In her analysis of the role of feeding work by Australian nurses in World War I, Harris (2015) argues that "providing food for health and recovery was a most important role for nurses" (p. 109). Rae (2005) maintains that the scarcity of food for troops, refugees, and the nurses themselves in certain war zones in World War I was so much that nurses sent food parcels to each other and officers brought food stuffs back from leave in Egypt, but there was little official response to the need. In their cultural history of food and war, Wood and Knight (2015) suggest that food was vital, not only to actual life but also to our understandings of life worth living.

Furthermore, they argue, in the hostile environment of World War I, food served as a link to home and safety.

There is a considerable amount of literature that points to the importance of nurses working as valued providers of food in war, but much of it relates to World War I rather than World War II. However, World War II is important to consider as it was the first truly mobile war and more like modern conflict than the wars previous to it. The movement of patients and personnel across large spaces, such as through the deserts of North Africa or the islands of Southeast Asia, meant that access to food during mobilization was frequently limited. Patients often arrived at hospitals severely malnourished, and distances across many war zones prevented sufficient food stuffs being provided to hospitals themselves for these patients in need. Also, because of the totality of World War II, the conflict gave rise to large numbers of refugees and interned civilians, again very much like current conflicts across the globe. Recent media coverage of civilians, including children starving in the Middle East and the aid agencies facing difficulties in getting food to these people, highlights the importance of nutrition in modern war. Consideration of the patient-feeding work of nurses in World War II would therefore appear to offer a critical contribution to the writings of wartime nursing work.

There are, however, a few exceptions to the limited discussions of the nurses' patient-feeding work in World War II. Within these explorations, there are some useful analyses of the challenges that nurses faced and how they overcame them. Brooks (2015) argues elsewhere that the lack of understanding by military personnel of the nutritional needs of the mainly Jewish inmates after years of starvation led to thousands of deaths in the early weeks following the liberation of Bergen-Belsen in April 1945. However, as knowledge of the dangers of overfeeding the starving was realized, the nurses, through kindness and patience, were able not only to support the improved nutritional status of the former inmates, but also to support their mental rehabilitation and return to humanity through mealtime ritual (Brooks, 2015). The involvement of British military nurses in caring for Polish refugees, many of whom were riddled with typhus and suffering from starvation, also identifies that where there is a limited arsenal of treatments available, the provision of nutritious food is vital to return the population to health. Thus, "at the combined hospital in Persia, the patients were fed three times per day"—a combination of stew, bread, eggs, and puddings (Brooks, 2014, p. 1514). Toman (2007) acknowledges the importance of nutrition to the war nurses' work, but does not elaborate on that importance, stating that the nurses on active service overseas considered it part of "real nursing things" (p. 153).

The one environment in which military nurses' feeding work is consistently mentioned in World War II literature is within discussions of life in the internment camps under Japanese occupation, although even this is not extensive. Twomey (2009) identifies the limited food available, but does not offer any analysis of how nurses or others managed this. Evans (2013) argues that the food in Changi Prison was inadequate to maintain health and well-being, except during July and August 1945. All prisoners, therefore, suffered from malnutrition, beriberi, dysentery, edema, and tropical ulcers—diseases also prevalent in combatants of all nationalities in Southeast Asia, Africa, and the Middle East. In many other camps, although the provision of food was not extensive at any time, it worsened as the war progressed. At Santo Tomas Internment Camp in Manila, the nurses were able to plant a small garden containing vegetables rich in vitamins and essential minerals to supplement the poorly balanced diet provided by the Japanese. Such inventiveness enabled them to save a number of lives, and "the internees undeniably benefitted from the nurses' expertise" (Kaminski, 2000, p. 90), although those older than 50 years did not fare well (Norman & Eifried, 1995, p. 117). Archer and Fedorowich (1996) consider the diet kitchens for infants and children that were established by the nurses at Stanley Camp on Hong Kong Island, but admit that the nurses found it difficult to provide the food that was needed. According to Bassett (1992), the Australian nurses also planted a vegetable garden in order to try to provide sufficient food, but once the vegetables were ready for harvesting, the Japanese took them.

Although this brief review does demonstrate some consideration of the importance of food and feeding to nurses' work in time of war, it does suggest rather limited discussions. This is in stark contrast to the extensive descriptions in military nurses' personal testimonies of food, feeding, and the attempts to prevent starvation and restore health in World War II. The primary data point to this as work that the nurses considered essential to the war effort and that contributed to a significant part of their working day, yet it was continuously challenged by the exigencies and environment of war. The chapter, therefore, now examines some of the primary data of nursing work in World War II. Focusing on the example of feeding work, it demonstrates the abilities of nurses in war to innovate and improvise to provide care and support for their ill and injured patients.

CASE STUDY: "There Were Definite Cases of Malnutrition"

Sister Jessie Wilson (n.d.) described how, in her tented hospital in Greece, they had 39 patients to a tent and no orderly. All the men were exhausted from battle and needed hygiene care, dressing changes, and feeding. There was no hot water or kitchen available in the tented hospital and so everything had to be carried by hand to the hospital from a nearby hotel; even the matron made "huge jugs of soup, and carried then up the hill to the hospital" (Wilson, p. 17). The involvement of the most senior nurse in the hospital in the feeding of combatant patients illustrates the criticality of this aspect of nursing work for injured and battle-exhausted men. The realization of the effects of battle exhaustion meant that nurses soon learned it was not only the physical need for food that demanded highly skilled nursing, but also the psychological improvements that could be garnered through the nurses' empathy. In October 1943, Sister A. K. D. Morgan (1943) was caring for the troops in Italy and had on her ward a young soldier of only 19 years. He did not, she wrote to her mother, "like any or all of the drinks and jellies and all the things we perjure our souls to procure for him, but mutters in a little weak voice, 'me [sic] mother makes OXO for me when I feel sick at home'" (p. 231). For those men, traumatized by war and suffering from what was known commonly as "shell shock," feeding took on a particular importance, requiring gentleness and patience (Morris, n.d., p. 152). However, Sister Mary Morris realized that patient feeding can also act as a form of occupational therapy for those suffering from trauma, as she watched one shell-shocked patient feed another patient who was blind. "I have asked Lt. Martin to take care of feeding him. He shakes far less now" (Morris, p. 120).

The importance, therefore, of not only the physical benefits of food, but also the psychological benefits of patient support

(continued)

CASE STUDY: "There Were Definite Cases of Malnutrition" *(continued)*

were understood by Morris as she cared for her combatant patients. The need for such tender ministrations, she acknowledged, was despite the apparent futility of "repairing their bodies so that they will be fit enough to go back to the front and fight all over again" (Morris, n.d., p. 167). She also appreciated the innovative and perhaps somewhat radical approach to her patient care when she wrote, "I call it 'patient participation,' but I dare not imagine what Matron will say when she finds out" (Morris, p. 110). In the later months of the war, when she was caring for released prisoners of war (POWs) in Belgium, she recalled: "Large numbers of our men, after years of captivity and semi-starvation, had fallen to tuberculosis and other illnesses. There were cases of definite malnutrition—these required very careful feeding" (Morris, p. 68). Sister Helen Luker (n.d.) also noted the particular needs of POWs after years in captivity, acknowledging both the great value placed on the food sent by the Red Cross and the employment of a catering officer who could improve the variety of food available after years of deprivation (p. 15). Her acknowledgment of the care and thought required in the feeding of those suffering from malnutrition demonstrates the importance and skill of this work— work that remained a key aspect of war nursing for nurses in all the war zones.

Sisters Edith Stevenson and Muriel Bostock were evacuated from Singapore in February 1942 on the *SS Heather,* a small hospital boat, little more than a tanker. They were specifically taken in order to care for patients on the ship where their scientific nursing understanding of caring for nutritionally depleted patients came to the fore:

> Our patients had travelled by various routes, up rivers, through jungle and mosqueto [*sic*] infected area, some already had maleria [*sic*] and dysentry [*sic*] and there were a lot of eye infections, ulcers on legs from leech bites and infection which were the

(continued)

CASE STUDY: "There Were Definite Cases of Malnutrition" *(continued)*

> result of walking through swamps. Lack of food
> also added to their debilitated condition. (Stevenson,
> 1994, p. 23)

Stevenson, Bostock, and their patients were fortunate to have
been evacuated on a ship that escaped to Sri Lanka successfully, enabling them to be admitted to hospitals away from
occupied lands. For those who were captured, the years under
occupation and in camps took their toll. Sister Dorothy Ingram
was a POW in Hong Kong from Christmas 1941 to September
1945. Her memoir offers stark descriptions of the levels of malnutrition, but also the collegiality and ingenuity of the nurses.
By February 1942, only 2 months following capitulation, there
were growing concerns about how to feed the patients with
dysentery. In order to deal with the problem, a meeting was held
between the matron and the Army and Navy commanding
officers (Ingram, n.d., p. 5). Given the importance placed on
nutrition by the most senior medical and nursing staff, it was
incumbent on all the nurses in captivity to improvise and innovate as required in order to provide the best food possible for
their patients. Nevertheless, as the occupation of Hong Kong
progressed, the limited access to food became a serious problem and Ingram and her colleagues needed to use all their
ingenuity to provide even a semblance of a balanced diet.
Despite the ongoing extreme difficulties in finding sufficient
food, the nurses used their resourcefulness to provide what
nourishment they could for their patients:

> I also worked in a malnutrition clinic twice a week
> and gave injections of Vitamin B, as many people got
> beri-beri. To try and cure eye trouble, soya bean milk
> was given. To provide Vitamin C we were encour-
> aged to make pine needle tea. (Ingram, n.d., p. 7)

DISCUSSION AND CONCLUSION

The nurses who went on active service overseas during World War II demonstrated that they could use their ingenuity to improvise and innovate and thus support the healing and recovery of combatants, who could then be returned to the battlefield. The ethical significance of patching up soldiers to return them to potential life-changing injury or death was obvious to the British nurses and their Allied nursing colleagues. The contradictions inherent in being a member of a healing profession and also being part of the war effort were not lost on the majority of nursing staff. Yet, they realized that the war would occur with them as part of it, or not, and as Sister Penny Salter (n.d.) argued with a military policeman in Burma, when he suggested that the so-called Valley of Death was no place for a woman, "But surely someone has to nurse the troops, and who better than us?" (p. 120). For those nurses who cared for civilians in internment camps under Japanese occupation, the situation was even worse. They had little access to the outside world and had only the resources that their captors provided, or those that they improvised for themselves. This chapter argues that despite the ethical and gendered difficulties of nurses' position in war zones, they demonstrated to their male superiors and themselves that they were expert practitioners. Through the focus on a traditional aspect of nursing work, that of patient feeding, the chapter identifies that the military nurses in World War II developed critical skills of innovation, improvisation, and ingenuity so necessary in a war that rendered them essential professionals in a war zone. Their stories act as a reminder that the role of the nurse in war is complex and diverse, and often ethically fraught. They also remind us that even a seemingly everyday task such as feeding was seen by nurses as an essential skill, requiring scientific and technical expertise, and an integral part of the war effort.

ACTIVITIES FOR TEACHING AND LEARNING

This chapter reflected on the ethics and work undertaken by nurses who participated in World War II. The potential contradictions of professionals, dedicated to healing who then enter into a world of killing and maiming, were considered. The other aspect of this chapter was the expertise of military nurses in ensuring that their injured, diseased, and malnourished patients receive adequate nutrition when that may not be easily available.

1. Do you think that military nurses can participate in war and not be politically involved in the conflict?
2. What other expertise do you think that military nurses bring to a war zone?
3. What areas of expertise do you think military nurses have brought back from wars into civilian practice and have their civilian colleagues appreciated this expertise?

REFERENCES

Archer, B., & Fedorowich, K. (1996). The women of Stanley: Internment in Hong Kong, 1942–45. *Women's History Review, 5*(3), 373–399.

Bassett, J. (1992). *Guns and brooches: Australian army nursing from the Boer War to the Gulf War*. Melbourne, Australia: Oxford University Press.

Brooks, J. (2014). Nursing typhus victims in the Second World War, 1942–1944. *Journal of Advanced Nursing, 70*(7), 1510–1519.

Brooks, J. (2015). "The nurse stoops down . . . for me": Nursing the liberated persons at Bergen-Belsen. In J. Brooks & C. E. Hallett (Eds.), *One hundred years of wartime nursing practices, 1854–1953* (pp. 211–231). Manchester, England: Manchester University Press.

Brooks, J., & Hallett, C. E. (2015). Introduction: The practice of nursing and the exigencies of war. In J. Brooks & C. E. Hallett (Eds.), *One hundred years of wartime nursing practices, 1854–1953* (pp. 1–19). Manchester, England: Manchester University Press.

Brown, K. (2008). *Fighting fit: Health, medicine and war in the twentieth century*. Stroud, England: The History Press [kindle edition].

Dale, C. (2015). Traversing the veldt with "Tommy Atkins": The clinical challenges of nursing typhoid patients during the Second Anglo-Boer War (1899–1902). In J. Brooks & C. E. Hallett (Eds.), *One hundred years of wartime nursing practices, 1854–1953* (pp. 58–77). Manchester, England: Manchester University Press.

D'Antonio, P. (2002). Nurses in war. *The Lancet, 360*(Suppl.), s7–s8.

Dixon Vuic, K. (2010). *Officer, nurse, woman: The Army Nurse Corps in the Vietnam War*. Baltimore, MD: Johns Hopkins University Press.

Elliot, B. (2015). Military nurses' experiences returning from war. *Journal of Advanced Nursing, 71*(5), 1066–1075.

Enloe, C. (1988). *Does khaki become you? The militarization of women's lives.* London, England: Pandora.

Evans, S. (2013). Culinary imagination as a survival tool: Ethel Mulvany and the Changi jail prisoners of war cookbook, Singapore, 1942–1945. *Canadian Military History, 22*(1), 39–49.

Finnegan, A., Finnegan, S., McKenna, H., McGhee, S., Ricketts, L., McCourt, K., . . . Thomas, M. (2016). Characteristics and values of British military nurse. International implications of war zone qualitative research. *Nurse Education Today, 36,* 86–95.

Griffiths, L., & Jasper, M. (2007). Warrior nurse: Duality and complementarity of role in the operational environment. *Journal of Advanced Nursing, 61*(1), 92–99.

Hallett, C. E. (2009). *Containing trauma: Nursing work in the First World War.* Manchester, England: Manchester University Press.

Hallett, C. E. (2014). *Veiled warriors: Allied nurses of the First World War.* Oxford, England: Oxford University Press.

Harris, K. (2015). "Health, healing and harmony": Invalid cookery and feeding by Australian nurses in the Middle East in the First World War. In J. Brooks & C. E. Hallett (Eds.), *One hundred years of wartime nursing practices, 1854–1953* (pp. 101–121). Manchester, England: Manchester University Press.

Harrison, M. (2004). *Medicine and victory: British military medicine in the Second World War.* Oxford, England: Oxford University Press.

Helmstadter, C. (2015). Class, gender and professional expertise: British military nursing in the Crimean War. In J. Brooks & C. E. Hallett (Eds.), *One hundred years of wartime nursing practices, 1854–1953* (pp. 23–41). Manchester, England: Manchester University Press.

Henderson, V. A. (1969). *Basic principles of nursing care.* Basel, Switzerland: S. Karger.

Ingram, Sister D. (nee de Wart). (n.d.). Experiences of an Army nurse: POW with Japanese. Imperial War Museums (Private Papers 93/18/1), London, England.

Kaminski, T. (2000). *Prisoners in paradise: American women in the wartime South Pacific.* Lawrence: University of Kansas Press.

Luker, Sister E. H. A. (n.d.). Diaries from 1940–45. Imperial War Museums (Private Papers 87/9/1), London, England.

Meehan, T. C. (2003). Careful nursing: A model for contemporary nursing practice. *Journal of Advanced Nursing, 44*(1), 99–107.

Morgan, A. K. D. (1943). Letter 65 (October): My dearest mums. Still with the lamp: Letters to my mother by an army nursing sister. Egypt—North Africa—Sicily—Italy, 1941–1944. Imperial War Museums (Private Papers 08/134/1), London, England.

Morris, M. (n.d.). Diary: Vol. 1. Imperial War Museums (Private Papers 80/38/1), London, England.

Nightingale, F. (1969). *Notes on nursing: What it is and what it is not.* New York, NY: Dover Publications [an unabridged republication of the first (1860) American edition].

Norman, E. M., & Eifried, S. (1995). How did they all survive? An analysis of American nurses' experiences in Japanese prisoner-of-war camps. *Nursing History Review, 3,* 105–127.

Rae, R. (2005). *Scarlet poppies: The army experience of Australian nurses during World War One.* Burwood, Australia: The College of Nursing.

Salter, Sister P. (n.d.). Long ago and far away: A distant memory. I am indebted to Maggie Burtenshaw and Dee Featherstone for providing me with Penny Salter's (whose real name was Muriel Kathleen Salter) diary. UK Centre for the History of Nursing and Midwifery, University of Manchester and Imperial War Museum, London, England, Documents, 17649.

Sarnecky, M. T. (1999). *A history of the U.S. Army Nurse Corps.* Philadelphia: University of Pennsylvania Press.

Starns, P. (2000). *Nurses at war: Women on the frontline, 1939–45.* Stroud, England: Sutton Publishing.

Stevenson, Sister E. (1994). The last lap: Autobiography 1912–1986. Imperial War Museums (Private Papers 86/29/1), London, England.

Toman, C. (2007). *An officer and a lady: Canadian military nursing and the Second World War.* Vancouver, BC, Canada: University of British Columbia Press.

Twomey, C. (2009). Double displacement: Western nurses return home from Japanese internment camps in Second World War. *Gender and History, 21*(3), 670–684.

Weeks-Shaw, C. (1902). *A text-book of nursing: For the use of training schools, families and private students.* New York, NY: Appleton.

Wilson, Sister J. S. C. (also known as Joan Katherine Wilson). (n.d.). We also served, 1940. . . . I am indebted to Jessie Wilson's family for providing me with access to this war diary. UK Centre for the History of Nursing and Midwifery, University of Manchester, England.

Wood, P. J., & Knight, S. (2015). The taste of war: The meaning of food to New Zealand and Australian nurses far from home in World War I, 1915–18. In G. M. Fealy, C. E. Hallett, & S. Malchau Dietz (Eds.), *Histories of nursing practice* (pp. 35–51). Manchester, England: Manchester University Press.

Chapter 5: Lives Not Worth Living: Ethical Dilemmas of Nursing in Nazi Germany

LINDA SHIELDS AND SUSAN BENEDICT

This process of degradation is progressive. You agree with a certain principle and you carry on in the same way without even letting yourself see where it's leading you. I'm sure all the terrible things done in the world begin with small acts of cowardice. (Ima Spanjaard, Auschwitz survivor, talking about the sterilization experiments).
(Shelley, 1991, p. 49)

Nurses today face a multitude of ethical issues in their practice: Are the elderly receiving optimal health care? Are they being restrained against their will? Are children able to have their parents with them during a hospital admission? Are medication errors reported appropriately? Are those from ethnic groups outside the mainstream able to receive equitable health care? These seem like everyday questions, but they are also deeply ethical ones and reach to the heart of nursing's legitimacy and its core premise of beneficence and nonmaleficence (American Nurses Association [ANA], 2015). Many nursing theorists remind us that we must be constantly alert to the inherent power that nursing has over other human beings, and alive to any sign of devaluation of humanity and human dignity (Holmes & Gastaldo, 2002; Perron, Fluet, & Holmes, 2005).

Contemporary nursing is now governed by a multitude of codes of ethics at both the global and local levels. The International Council of Nurses (ICN) developed its codes of ethics in 1953 and continually revises the document in order to respond to changing social norms and expanding concepts of human rights (ICN, 2012). These codes were developed largely as a result of changing social norms about human rights and the revelation of atrocities committed by medical professionals, including nurses, before and during World War II, in particular during the period known as the Third Reich, or "Nazi Germany." However, even in Nazi Germany such documents existed (Reich Circular of February 1931, in Grodin, 1992). The question for all who read this chapter is how nurses came to believe that killing their patients was a legitimate part of their nursing role. This is not a question that we can merely relegate to the past and dismiss as something that would not happen today. Stories of nurses in Nazi Germany resonate with many ongoing ethical and human rights issues evident across the world, and need to be taken seriously by nurses in practice today.

BACKGROUND

Nursing in Nazi Germany

Nursing and the Third Reich

Some nurses in the Nazi era before and during World War II were guilty of, and complicit in, crimes against humanity. Guided by Nazi philosophies and under pressure from the enormous propaganda machine that was an inherent part of the Nazi era, some nurses made the choice to kill their patients. This chapter describes these nurses, how they were influenced by Nazism, and the ethics of what they did. It also discusses a very courageous nurse who resisted and saved people. This demonstrates both sides of the ethical divide, which is relevant today with the plethora of ethical dilemmas for nurses.

Nurses, like other citizens of the Third Reich of Nazi Germany, came to accept that many lives were not perfect, for example, the disabled, who were described as "life not worth living" and thus not worth the support that the institutionally disabled required (Steppe, 1991, 1992). The Nazis believed that it was better to kill them and save the money (Benedict & Shields, 2014). People who did not fit a certain image of ethnic desirability—White, Nordic, Aryan—should be first excluded from society, then kept from reproducing, then isolated, and finally killed (Burleigh, 1994). Nurses were perpetrators in this process (Benedict & Shields, 2014). Nurses set aside their individual consciences as being inconsequential and adopted the mores of the government: The health of the individual was less important than the wellness of the *Volk*—the collective people—and "diseased" elements within the *Volk* should be eliminated. Nursing turned its view from the care of the individual to the care of the state with horrible consequences for all (Foth, 2013). Nurses and midwives were essential to the Nazi's plan for a healthy and racially pure state (McFarland-Icke, 1994). Much has been written about the roles and actions of the physicians in the killings under the "euthanasia"[1] programs and the medical experiments of the concentration camps, but, until recently, little has been written about the roles of nurses and midwives.

In the Nazi era, German nurses were similar in education and practice to other nurses in Western Europe and the United States. They cared for their patients and they underwent mainly hospital-based training of a high standard (Florence Nightingale herself went to Germany specifically to study nursing; Nelson & Rafferty, 2010); there was a range of specialties in which nurses could work and a range of nursing associations to which nurses had to belong. In addition to Red Cross nurses, there were Catholic nurses (the Caritas) and the Protestant nurses association (*Diakoniegemeinschaft*). There were the free nurses who did not belong to any of the religious organizations, and a small group of Jewish nurses. In 1934, the National Socialist Nurses' Organization—known as the "Brown Sisters" because of their brown uniforms—was formed (Lagerway, 2006). These nurses were educated according to the principles of National Socialism and swore an oath of allegiance to Hitler, as did the nurses of the Red Cross.

Nursing During the "Euthanasia" Program

A particular focus of much of this research about nurses and midwives has been on the so-called "euthanasia" programs in which disabled children and adults who were institutionalized were killed (Benedict & Kuhla, 1999). Although couched in the cover story that the hospital beds and personnel were needed for Germany's war-wounded, the true

---

1. In line with common practice, we place the word "euthanasia" in quotes to demonstrate that in the Nazi context, this was a misnomer. Euthanasia means a good death, and there was nothing good about how these people were killed. The word "euthanasia" was chosen by the Nazis to promote murder as mercy killing (Burleigh, 1994).

underlying rationale was the belief that the disabled were of no value—
they were called "useless eaters"—and, furthermore, were a danger to
the health of the German people who could be "contaminated" by these
"inferior" genes. This key principle of National Socialism, racial hygiene,
started with laws preventing marriage between ethnic Germans and
people of "inferior" races, then involuntary sterilization of people with
disabilities, and the eventual killing of the disabled (Burleigh, 1994).

The killing of disabled children started before the adult "eutha-
nasia" programs and continued unabated throughout World War II
(Benedict, O'Donnell, & Shields, 2009). However, the killing of adult
patients had two separate and distinct phases. The first, known as
Aktion T-4, for the address of its organizational headquarters at
Tiergartenstrasse 4 in Berlin, involved establishing a total of six killing
centers at psychiatric hospitals: Bernburg, Brandenburg, Grafeneck,
Hadamar, Hartheim, and Sonnenstein (Figure 5.1; Benedict, 2014a;
Burleigh, 1994). Each of these had a gas chamber and groups of patients
were killed together. Patients from throughout the Reich were transported to these centers to be gassed. Nurses did not kill the patients

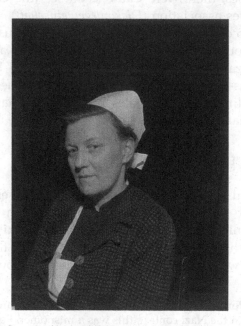

FIGURE 5.1 Portrait of Irmgard Huber, one of the chief nurses at Hadamar
Psychiatric Hospital, a main "euthanasia" killing center.
Source: United States Holocaust Memorial Museum Archives, #05469.

in this phase; however, they were complicit. They helped ready the patients for the trips to the killing centers, rode with them on the buses, assisted with undressing them, and escorted them to the gas chambers. Finally, the nurses rode back to their home institutions with the now deceased patients' belongings. This phase of the "euthanasia" program continued until August 1941. Knowledge of the killings became widespread and was condemned by many, thus the gassings stopped; however, the killing of the disabled continued but on an individual basis and usually by fatal overdoses of drugs. This phase of killing the disabled was known as "wild euthanasia" or "decentralized euthanasia" because patients were killed in many hospitals throughout Germany and occupied territories. In this phase of the "euthanasia program," it was usually the physicians who designated which patients were to be killed but it was the nurses who did the actual killings (Benedict et al., 2009; Burleigh, 1994).

Nurses in the Death Camps and the Concentration Camps

Preceding and during World War II, the Germans established concentration camps to house not only criminals but also hundreds of thousands of people who were deemed to be enemies of the Reich or who were members of ethnic groups thought to be "inferior" or threats to the state (Burleigh, 1994). Among these were Jews, Jehovah's Witnesses, homosexuals, and Roma and Sinti (so-called "Gypsies"). Although most of these camps were established as labor camps, others—Chelmo, Belzec, Sobibor, Treblinka, Auschwitz/Birkenau, and Madjanek—were death camps; that is, camps whose sole purpose was the murder of certain groups of people (Sereny, 1974). The murder of millions of Jews from all over Europe was known as the "Final Solution" and is known today as the "Holocaust" or the "Shoah." In the death camps of Treblinka, Sobibor, and Belzec, male nurses who had perfected their killing skills in the T-4 "euthanasia" program were brought in to establish and run, along with other men, the gas chambers that had been perfected during the "euthanasia" program (Sereny, 1974). In other concentration camps, hundreds of thousands of prisoners died; however, death was considered by the Nazis merely an acceptable by-product, whereas slave labor was the primary intent. In these camps, there were hospitals that were staffed by either nurses who were prisoners, or those employed by the *Schutzstaffel* or SS (Benedict et al., 2009).

In many of the concentration camps, horrific medical experiments were carried out on the prisoners (Benedict, 2003; Strzelecka, 2000;

Weindling, 2004). In general, these experiments can be categorized into experiments related to war and experiments related to racial hygiene. Nurses participated in both. Prisoners were used as "lab rats," had no way of giving consent, and, if they survived the experiments—thousands did not—were killed afterward in the gas chambers. Nurses helped in the wards, held people down (often no anesthetic was used and usually no pain relief was given), prepared them for surgery, helped with x-rays used for sterilization, and so forth.

No one was forced to be part of the crimes of the "euthanasia" programs of Nazi Germany, although there was putative duress. There is no record of "a single case that someone who refused to participate in killing operations was shot, incarcerated, or penalized" (Friedlander, 1995, p. 235). Similar to the men who were members of the *Einsatzgruppen* (Browning, 1998), the specialized killing units who went into the countries occupied by Nazi Germany specifically to round up and shoot all the Jews, nurses who worked in the "euthanasia" programs could refuse to be involved and they likely would be moved to another ward or another hospital, although there are reports that some requests were denied (Sagel-Grande, Fuchs, & Reuter, 1979). Others were successful, for example, Elly Büchsenschuss, who worked as a caregiver at the psychiatric hospital at Meseritz-Obrawalde (Büchsenschuss, 1962). In other words, the nurses who participated in these crimes did so either because they believed that they were relieving patients of their suffering, because they believed in the importance and necessity of their mission, or because of alleged duress. Others, when questioned at trials, gave more mundane reasons, such as needing to keep their jobs; however, there were some nurses who held to their codes of ethics and took extremely courageous risks to save people. The case studies in this chapter provide examples of both situations.

CASE STUDY: Antonia Pachner

Antonia Pachner was head nurse at the *Siechenhaus*[1] in the psychiatric institution at Klagenfurt in Austria (Benedict, 2014b). People were admitted there if they had a mental illness or a learning disability. In 1946, Pachner was hanged for killing at

(continued)

CASE STUDY: Antonia Pachner *(continued)*

least 20 of her patients. Accurate numbers will never be known because, while the deaths were recorded, the causes of death were inaccurately stated to be natural causes rather than "homicide." Why did a qualified nurse, educated in the standards of nursing and midwifery of the time, come to kill? Some of her answers at her trial give us an idea.

> I am aware that the killing of patients is against the law and is not something any caregiver should see as within her duties. I am unable to explain why I did not refuse Dr. Niedermoser's orders. I think I was afraid of being dismissed. . . . For killings of the infants and small children, I did have general orders from Dr. Niedermoser. I never liked to do the killings but had to do them when Dr. Niedermoser explained to me that this or that patient needed to be killed. (Pachner, 1945)

Apart from the obvious conclusion that Pachner committed murder, it seems that she saw this as a part of her daily duties.

---

1. *Siechenhaus* is a term that is no longer in common use. The original meaning could best be translated as "old folks' home." Comparable units are now referred to as geriatric units. Patients could be directly admitted to the *Siechenhaus* without being patients in the hospital. These were the "frail elderly" or those who otherwise could not care for themselves (Benedict, 2014b, p. 162).

CASE STUDY: Maria Stromberger

Maria Stromberger, a nurse from Austria, applied for a transfer to Auschwitz so that she could provide care to prisoner patients (Figure 5.2). This was not allowed, however, because

(continued)

CASE STUDY: Maria Stromberger *(continued)*

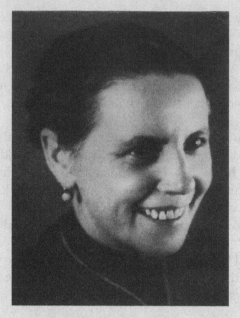

FIGURE 5.2 Maria Stromberger.
Courtesy of Archiv der Landeshauptstadt Bregenz.

only prisoner nurses and prisoner physicians could provide care in the camp's hospital, so Stromberger was assigned to the hospital for the SS soldiers stationed at Auschwitz where she began work as the *Oberschwester* (head nurse) in October 1942. By that time, Auschwitz was fully functioning as a death factory to kill Jews and others considered dispensable by the Nazi state. The SS hospital was located near the gas chambers in Auschwitz and Stromberger was able to see the prisoners lined up to be killed (Benedict, 2006).

During the 2-1/2 years she worked there, she smuggled food and medicine to prisoners, and was able to clandestinely bring guns into the camp for the Polish Resistance. More importantly, she smuggled out letters, diaries, and undeveloped photographs, which the Resistance collected from prisoners.

(continued)

CASE STUDY: Maria Stromberger (continued)

Stromberger delivered these items to members of the Austrian Resistance on her many trips outside of Auschwitz.

It is hard for anyone to imagine what Maria Stromberger did and the risks she took. If she had been caught, she would have instantly been killed, but she was never found out. It is easy to hope that in a similar situation, one would act as courageously as she did; however, it is impossible to say what one would do in such circumstances. Maria Stromberger stands as an important role model for all nurses today.

DISCUSSION AND CONCLUSION

Information about the Holocaust and the role of nurses in the Nazi crimes are rarely found in nursing curricula (Shields, Hartin, Shields, & Benedict, 2015). Nonetheless, it is an important way to teach nurses about ethics and how the situations in which they find themselves can be at the top of a slippery slope of dilemma and complex decision making. Possibly the most extreme example of this today is the involvement of nurses in executions in countries where capital punishment is lawful (Hinojosa, 2006; Hooten & Shipman, 2013).

As nursing as a profession comes to grips with this emerging field of scholarship, more details will emerge of nurses involved in war crimes. These studies will not be limited to the Nazi era. The role of nurses in the horrific medical experiments in Japanese camps in China in the 1930s is yet to be examined, and in more recent times, nurses have been complicit in atrocities such as the Rwandan genocide (African Rights, 1995). These, too, need detailed examination.

With the examples of Antonia Pachner and Maria Stromberger, we present two extremes. On the one hand, we have the criminal nurse who believed that killing her patients was a part of her caring role. On the other hand, we find a heroine whose actions put her in grave danger each day but she persisted because she believed that what she was doing was the right thing. It is (hopefully) unlikely that readers of this book will find themselves in such extreme situations as Pachner and Stromberger; however, in more recent times, similar things have occurred. Nurses were involved in the killings in the Rwandan geno-cide (African Rights, 1995) and, in countries that support capital punish-ment, nurses insert the intravenous lines through which lethal drugs are given (Hinojosa, 2006, Hooten & Shipman, 2013). Nurses force-fed prisoners at Guantanamo Bay (ANA, 2016; Boivin, 2006) and continue to staff the health services in Australia's off-shore immigration deten-tion centers, where even children are incarcerated (McCann et al., 2014). These are many examples of nurses abrogating their codes of ethics (ANA, 2010; ICN, 2012) as well as acting in unethical and morally wrong ways. History is an important teacher, and it is imperative that nurses know what people like Antonia Pachner did, as well as the heroic actions of nurses such as Maria Stromberger, so that they can make informed and morally right decisions when faced with the ethical dilemmas with which modern nursing practice abounds.

Nurses are in a privileged position. They have the right to give care to those who need it in what are often the most vulnerable parts of their lives. Therefore, nurses have a responsibility to ensure their practice is as ethical as possible. It is incumbent on all who take on this role to understand what the nurses in Nazi Germany did—how they were influenced by Nazi philosophies, how they made their decisions relating to their nursing practice, and how they came to believe that killing was a legitimate part of their caring role. If one reads the inter-view of the nurse who helps with insertion of intravenous lines for lethal injections, one is struck by the similarities between the 2013 interview (Hinojosa, 2006) and the transcripts of trials of the convicted nurse perpetrators of Nazi Germany in regard to the reasoning and language used (Benedict & Shields, 2014). Only if today's nurses under-stand the decisions made by the nurses of the Nazi era, can they make balanced, ethical, and informed decisions about the patients in their care.

ACTIVITIES FOR TEACHING AND LEARNING

When answering these questions, reflect not only on what nurses did because of the conditions of the day, but also on today's nursing practice.

1. How and why did killing become just "routine"?
2. What was there in these nurses that they accepted this mission to kill their patients?

3. What education was available about ethics for nurses?
4. How did the Nazi ideologies come to be acceptable even though they negated everything that nurses had been taught to believe?
5. Note the fact that nurses had some qualms about killing adults, but none about killing infants. Why was this acceptable?
6. What made Maria Stromberger so different?
7. What would you do?

REFERENCES

African Rights. (1995). *Rwanda: Not so innocent: When women become killers.* Kigali, Rwanda: Author.

American Nurses Association. (2010). *Nurses' role in capital punishment.* ANA Center for Ethics and Human Rights. Retrieved from http://www.nursing world.org/MainMenuCategories/EthicsStandards/Ethics-Position-State ments/prtetcptl14447.pdf

American Nurses Association. (2015). *Code of ethics for nurses.* ANA Center for Ethics and Human Rights. Retrieved from http://www.nursingworld.org/ MainMenuCategories/EthicsStandards/CodeofEthicsforNurses

American Nurses Association. (2016). *Force-feeding of detainees at Guantanamo Bay.* ANA Center for Ethics and Human Rights. Retrieved from http://www .nursingworld.org/MainMenuCategories/EthicsStandards/Resources/ Force-feeding-of-Detainees-at-Guantanamo-Bay.html

Benedict, S. (2003). The nadir of nursing: Nurse-perpetrators of the Ravensbrück Concentration Camp. *Nursing History Review, 11,* 129–146.

Benedict, S. (2006). Maria Stromberger: A nurse in the resistance in Auschwitz. *Nursing History Review, 14,* 189–202.

Benedict, S. (2014a). The medicalization of murder: The "euthanasia" programs. In S. Benedict & L. Shields (Eds.), *Nurses and midwives in Nazi Germany: The "euthanasia programs"* (pp. 71–104). New York, NY: Routledge Studies in Modern European History.

Benedict, S. (2014b). Klagenfurt: "She killed as part of her daily duties." In S. Benedict & L. Shields (Eds.), *Nurses and midwives in Nazi Germany: The "euthanasia programs"* (pp. 140–163). New York, NY: Routledge Studies in Modern European History.

Benedict S., & Kuhla, J. (1999). Nurses' participation in the euthanasia programs of Nazi Germany. *Western Journal of Nursing Research, 21,* 246–263.

Benedict, S., O'Donnell, A., & Shields, L. (2009). Children's "euthanasia" in Nazi Germany. *Journal of Pediatric Nursing, 24*, 506–516. doi:10.1016/j.pedn .2008.07.012

Benedict, S., & Shields, L. (Eds.). (2014). *Nurses and midwives in Nazi Germany: The "euthanasia" programs.* New York, NY: Routledge History.

Boivin, J. (2014). Viewpoint: Nurse's refusal to force feed Gitmo prisoners triggers debate. *American Nurse Today, 9.* Retrieved from http://www.american nursetoday.com/viewpoint-nurses-refusal-force-feed-gitmo-prisoners-trig gers-debate

Browning, C. R. (1998). *Ordinary men—Reserve Battalion 101 and the final solution in Poland.* New York, NY: HarperCollins.

Burleigh, M. (1994). *Death and deliverance.* Cambridge, England: Cambridge University Press.

Büchsenschuss, E. (1962, May 28). *Testimony* (File no. 33.029/4). Staatarchiv München. Munich, Germany.

Foth, T. (2013). *Caring and killing: Nursing and psychiatric practice in Germany, 1931–1943.* Pflegewissenschaft und Pflegebildung. Göttingen, Germany: V&R unipress, Universität Osnabrück.

Friedlander, H. (1995). *The origins of Nazi genocide.* Chapel Hill, NC: University of North Carolina Press.

Grodin, M. (1992). Historical origins of the Nuremberg Code. In G. Annas & M. Grodin (Eds.), *The Nazi Doctors and the Nuremberg Code.* New York, NY: Oxford University Press.

Hinojosa, M. (2006). Web-extended interview: "Nurse Karen." Retrieved from http://www.pbs.org/now/shows/228/nurse-execution.html

Holmes, D., & Gastaldo, D. (2002). Nursing as means of governmentality. *Journal of Advanced Nursing, 38*(6), 557–565.

Hooten, J., & Shipman, D. (2013). Comment: The ethical dilemmas of nurses' participation in prisoner executions. *Nursing Ethics, 20*, 491–492. doi:10.1177/ 0969733013487821

International Council of Nurses (ICN). (2012). Torture, death penalty and participation by nurses in executions. Retrieved from http://www.icn.ch/ images/stories/documents/publications/position_statements/E13_Torture_ Death_Penalty_Executions.pdf

Lagerway, M. (2006). The Third Reich in the pages of the *American Journal of Nursing,* 1932–1950. *Nursing History Review, 14*, 59–87.

McCann, D., Dowden, S., Hutton, A., McNamara, J., Shields, L., et al. for Australian College of Children and Young People's Nurses. (2014). Position statement: Safeguarding the health of children seeking asylum in Australia. Retrieved from http://www.accypn.org.au/wp-content/uploads/220515_Position_Statement_Refugee_Children_Young_Peoples_Health.pdf

McFarland-Icke, B. (1999). *Nurses in Nazi Germany: Moral choice in history.* Princeton, NJ: Princeton University Press.

Nelson, S., & Rafferty, A-M. (2010). *Notes on Nightingale: The influence and legacy of a nursing icon.* Ithaca, NY: ILR Press.

Pachner, A. (1945, October 28). Arrest report. File obtained from *Dokumentationsarchiv des österreichischen Widerstandes* [Archives of the Austrian Resistance], Vienna, Austria.

Perron, A., Fluet, C., & Holmes, D. (2005). Agents of care and agents of the state: Bio-power and nursing practice. *Journal of Advanced Nursing, 50*(5), 536–544.

Sagel-Grande, I., Fuchs, H., & Reuter, C. (1979). Euthanasie Heil-und Pflegeanstalt Meseritz-Obrawalde, Lfd. 587, Vol. XX Sentencing from April 12, 1964–April 3, 1965. *Justiz und NS-Verbrechen.* Amsterdam, Netherlands: University of Amsterdam Press.

Sereny, G. (1974). *Into that darkness.* New York, NY: Vintage Books.

Shelley, L. (1991). *Criminal experiments on human beings in Auschwitz and war research laboratories: Twenty women prisoners' accounts.* San Francisco, CA: Mellen Research University Press.

Shields, L., Hartin, P., Shields, K., & Benedict, S. (2015). Teaching the Holocaust in nursing and medical education in Australia. *Working Papers in the Health Sciences, 1,* 1–4.

Steppe, H. (1991). Nursing in the Third Reich. *History of Nursing Society Journal, 3,* 21–37.

Steppe, H. (1992). Nursing in Nazi Germany. *Western Journal of Nursing Research, 14,* 744.

Strzelecka, I. (2000). Experiments. In W. Ditugoborski & F. Piper (Eds.), *Auschwitz 1940–1945* (Vol. 2). Oświęcim, Poland: Auschwitz-Birkenau State Museum.

Weindling, P. (2004). *Nazi medicine and the Nuremberg trials: From medical war crimes to informed consent.* Basingstoke, England: Palgrave MacMillan.

Section III: Mid-20th Century

Chapter 6: Toward Community-Based Practice: The Changing Role of the Registered Nurse in Psychiatry and Mental Health

KYLIE M. SMITH AND GEERTJE BOSCHMA

We were moving in the direction of psychotherapy. . . . We didn't call it that, we called it 1:1, and we called it "talking with patients" and then we called it counseling and then we called it therapy. That took from 1948 until 1960.

(Peplau, 1985)

The World Health Organization (WHO) was founded in 1946 and when members wrote its constitution they defined health as a "state of complete physical, mental and social well-being and not merely the absence of disease or infirmity" (WHO, 1946). In this immediate postwar period, mental health was considered just as important for social stability as physical health. In the decades that followed, the powerful rise of a biomedical approach to health resulted in a focus on the physical and disease aspects of human health, often to the detriment of mental and social well-being. However, since the early 1990s, mental health has been recognized as a global human rights issue, reinforced by the United Nations General Assembly with the adoption of principles for the protection of persons with mental illness and the improvement of mental health care (United Nations General Assembly, 1991). The adoption of these principles endorsed the need for the improvement of mental health services globally, and required that responses needed to become more effective and equitable. In response, the WHO developed several global strategies to enhance awareness of people's mental health needs, disseminate knowledge, and support policy to decrease inequities in service access for individuals and families with mental illness. In 2002, the WHO launched a global program, "Nations for Mental Health," with a particular focus on underserved populations. Major depression was identified as a leading cause of disability, among other illnesses such as epilepsy, schizophrenia, alcohol dependency, and the threat of suicide (Desjarlais, Eisenberg, Good, & Kleinman, 1995; WHO, 2002). Recognizing that for far too long mental health had been neglected, WHO argued in its final report on the topic that mental health was crucial to the overall well-being of individuals, societies, and countries. By the turn of the 21st century, mental health was recognized as a leading cause of disability and a priority health issue, globally. Nurses around the globe, united within the International Council of Nurses (ICN), advocated for national policies to ensure the breakdown of stigma and discrimination regarding mental health issues and to put in place more effective prevention and treatment programs (ICN, 2008; Saxena & Barrett, 2007).

How to best provide care and services to people affected by mental illness continues to be a pressing issue. In fact, many questions we face today are not new. Throughout the 20th century, health professionals and patients alike have argued for better mental health care, although insights on how such improvement should take place have fluctuated as cultural and social perceptions of mental illness have changed (Tomes, 2006). This chapter addresses two major shifts in mental health policy during the 20th century that have affected mental health practice and transformed the way nurses provide mental health service today. Firstly, we examine how advancement in nursing education and psychiatric theory generated new therapeutic work and new roles for nurses as clinical nurse specialists (Case Study I). Secondly, we discuss how mental health care shifted from a dominant context of institutional and mainly custodial care in the first half of the 20th century to a community-based practice, bringing new roles for nurses following World War II (Case Study II). These shifts and changes are central to how we practice mental health care today and form key moments in understanding mental health nurses' continued responses to challenging issues of stigma, lack of service, and human rights. Historical knowledge of these changes provides the context by which to understand the direction of contemporary mental health nursing, especially as nurses seek to address new questions of scope of practice, consumer-driven care, and mental health promotion today.

BACKGROUND

This section sets out the background to developments in psychiatry that have shaped the nature of contemporary nursing practice, demonstrating how changes in science and medicine, and the shifting sands of politics and policies, have affected the development of nurse-specific theory and practice. By the end of World War I (1914–1918), hospitalization in large, state-funded mental hospitals was the dominant mode of psychiatric treatment. Such hospitals, mostly overcrowded and not providing much more than custodial care, became increasingly criticized for their inadequacy, especially when war veterans suffering from shell shock returned home to find there was little help available for them (D'Antonio, 2006; Grob, 1994). New scientific insights on prevention within an emerging mental hygiene movement gained momentum (Boschma, 2012). However, the impact of economic depression in the 1930s impeded efforts of change and reform.

Sweeping changes moved through psychiatry and psychology in the decades on either side of World War II, which came to profoundly affect nursing. American psychiatry lagged "behind" European practice in that there was no coherent, evidence-based approach to psychiatric theory, practice, or science in the early 20th century, which concerned practitioners in the politically tense era just prior to World War II (Deutsch, 1937; Grinker & Speigel, 1945; Menninger, 1948; Rees, 1945). In the absence of any real successful "medicine," psychiatry as a profession in the United States in particular, was in desperate need of scientific and professional legitimacy (Dowbiggin, 1997; Grob, 1991; Pressman, 1998). With the persecution of the Jews in Europe and the consequent diaspora, Freudian psychoanalysis began to have an impact in the United States after it had already begun to wane in Europe. Psychoanalysis found traction largely because it appeared to offer a way forward from moral treatment and mental hygiene, for it relied on theory and technique that needed to be learned (and learned a specific way). It offered structure and theory that appeared to explain cause and effect, and it offered something for psychiatrists to *do* that set them apart from neurologists (Grob, 1994; Hale, 1995; Lieberman, 2015).

For many practitioners emerging from the experience of World War II in particular, psychoanalysis was seen as a useful tool because their wartime experience had led them to focus on mental illness that could be categorized as neurosis, which they believed was caused by environmental factors and could be treated. This concept of illness as behavioral rather than purely biological was the subject of much debate in Western psychiatry after World War II (Grob, 1991). In the United States, the Group for the Advancement of Psychiatry (GAP), led by William Menninger, engaged in a protracted struggle to wrestle mental health away from a strictly biomedical model to a more psychotherapeutic one, and this influence on public thinking and policy at this time was profound (Deutsch, 1959; Grob, 1991, 1994). These events occurred in the context of a rapidly changing policy and practice environment in the United States after World War II, where the passing of the National Mental Health Act in 1946 released vast amounts of funding for the establishment of the National Institute of Mental Health (NIMH) and the development of advanced educational programs for the mental health professions, including nursing. Historian Gerald Grob has suggested that nurses were not particularly vocal or active within psychiatry at this time due to the lack of numbers in the specialty, high turnover rates due to marriage, and the absence of any nursing scholarship (Grob, 1991, pp. 118–119). While these points are arguable, Grob is correct to the extent that nurses were largely perceived as under the control of the broader psychiatric hierarchy (Grob, 1991, p. 120). As had been the case for the medical profession before it, psychiatry needed nurses to help with its image problem. If psychiatry was to be taken seriously as an institution-based "medical" science, rather than head shrinking quackery with dubious ethics and practiced in Bedlam-type asylums, then respectable, educated, and well-trained nurses were central to this project.

Recently, scholars have attempted to address the role of the nurse within the changing field of psychiatry, documenting the type of work and care that they undertook and how these roles changed as the profession of nursing came to impact ideas about institutional care (Borsay & Dale, 2015; Boschma, 2003, 2012, 2013; D'Antonio, 2004, 2006; D'Antonio, Beeber, Sills, & Nagle, 2014; Olson, 1996). Within this work, Olson (1996) has argued that the mid-20th century was an important but difficult time for North American nurses as they struggled to identify what was unique to their practice and argued about the place of mental health nursing as a specialty in nurse education. Olson demonstrates the centrality of the idea of interpersonal theory, which

D'Antonio et al. (2014) have argued has been overshadowed by "the biologically and specialty based imperatives that have subsumed the significance of relationships in our practice" (p. 312). D'Antonio et al. argue that there is much to be learned from mid-century psychiatric nurse theorists, who championed the idea of the therapeutic relationship as the essence of mental health nursing practice. Boschma's (2003) and Borsay and Dale's (2015) collections demonstrate how these changing ideas about the nature of psychiatric illness and its related treatments affected the professional identity and the type of paid work that attendants and nurses undertook in institutions in Europe, the United Kingdom, and Australia throughout the 19th and 20th centuries. These scholars show that although there were differences in the evolution of psychiatric nursing that were specific to time and place, mental health nursing followed the same trends as general nursing toward increasing specialization and professionalization. These trends were shaped by local culture and politics, and the ability of nursing as an emerging profession to advocate for its role within broader mental health policy.

Psychiatric nurse education therefore became a hotly contested subject. Although the field had initially developed within mental hospital-based training schools, which were modeled after similar examples in general hospitals, by the end of the 1940s such educational models no longer fit the need or the scope of mental health nursing practice and new knowledge was urgently needed. It was in the United States that the first attempt at establishing mental health nursing as an advanced practice specialization was undertaken, and this took the form of new graduate courses, run wholly by nurses, in universities. The Case Study I addresses this change, offering two examples from the U.S. context about the way the influential U.S. nurse leaders, Laura Wood Fitzsimmons and Hildegard Peplau, took on a leading role in this transformation.

CASE STUDY I: Establishing Graduate Courses in the United States

The efforts of nurses to develop advanced practice courses were predicated on the availability of funding and the work of specific nurse leaders who attempted to redefine the role of psychiatric nursing. This process had begun during World War II when the American Psychiatric Association (APA) had

(continued)

CASE STUDY I: Establishing Graduate Courses in the United States *(continued)*

acquired funding from the Rockefeller Foundation to establish a "nurse consultant" program. In 1941, the chair of the APA's Committee on Psychiatric Nursing, Charles Fitzpatrick, wrote to the Rockefeller Foundation about the "emergency" in the current psychiatric nursing situation and requested funding for the employment of a "nurse consultant" who could act as a liaison between the APA, nursing bodies such as the National League of Nursing Education (NLNE), and schools of nursing (Fitzpatrick, 1941). The Rockefellers agreed and in July 1942 the APA appointed Laura Wood Fitzsimmons, RN, as its inaugural nurse consultant. Fitzsimmons was born in Virginia and trained at Walter Reed Veterans Administration Hospital. She had served as an Army nurse and was awarded a BSc degree from Columbia University in 1938. She was superintendent of nursing at St. Elizabeth's Hospital, a psychiatric hospital in Washington, DC, when she came to work for the APA and the Rockefellers.

Fitzsimmons's first task was to conduct a survey of the state of the field, and she did this through written questionnaires and personal visits. She traveled across the United States and Canada and documented the state of psychiatric nursing workforces as well as systems for nurse education, which culminated in a report delivered to the APA and the Rockefeller Foundation in June 1944. The report made eight major recommendations for the postwar period. These included the need for public awareness campaigns about mental illness; an increase of funds into mental health so as to facilitate better standards of hours, wages, and conditions for workers; a uniform system of training for attendants; the development of uniform standards of care for patients; more clinical placements in mental health for student nurses; the improvement of schools of nursing associated with mental hospitals; the revival and expansion of postgraduate courses in mental health; the specific professional recognition for mental health nurses; and the organization of mental health staff under a director of nursing (Fitzsimmons, 1944a).

(continued)

CASE STUDY I: Establishing Graduate Courses in the United States *(continued)*

Although the APA was most interested in her work on attendants and aides training, Fitzsimmons herself was more concerned with the issue of education for nurses. Her work on attendants, culminating in a 371-page training manual, which the APA and Rockefellers printed and distributed to all North American psychiatric hospitals, had really sought to try and differentiate the nature of attendant or aide work from that of the RN (Figure 6.1).

Having dealt with that issue, Fitzsimmons moved her focus more intently to the development of university courses for psychiatric nursing. As Alan Gregg, the Rockefellers' director of medical services, noted in his diary in June 1945:

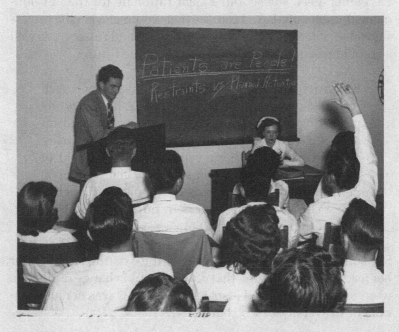

FIGURE 6.1 Bernard Hall, MD, and Esther Lazaro, RN, associate director, School for Psychiatric Aides, Winter Veterans Administration Hospital, Topeka, Kansas, 1949.
Source: Rockefeller Archive Center.

(continued)

CASE STUDY I: Establishing Graduate Courses in the United
States *(continued)*

> Mrs F-S says she wants next year's emphasis to be
> spent principally on the development of postgradu-
> ate courses in psychiatric nursing. . . . The desperately
> urgent need is for registered nurses with thorough
> postgraduate training in psychiatric nursing who
> can teach students and students of nursing on affili-
> ation. (Gregg, 1945)

If there were to be any meaningful development of psychiatric
nursing skills, then skilled nurses were needed to teach the next
generation. Fitzsimmons wrote publically about these issues
in journal articles. Writing in the *American Journal of Nursing* in
December 1944, she set out a clear rationale for the development of university-based courses that would elevate the profession into the realm of academic scholarship and research, as well
as provide leaders and administrators in the future:

> For years we have talked about the need for a well
> rounded program of nurse education yet, while
> preaching this doctrine, year after year hundreds of
> nurses have been graduated from schools of nursing
> without having had any experience in the field of
> psychiatric nursing while psychiatry claims over 50
> percent of the hospital beds of the nation. This has
> given concern to the leaders in nursing education.
> (Fitzsimmons, 1944b, p. 1166)

She summed up her 2-year survey of the existing situation for
her readers by explaining that nothing could change until there
were adequately trained instructors, and this was her justification for university-based courses:

> . . . little can be done to advance psychiatric train-
> ing at an undergraduate level . . . until more key

(continued)

CASE STUDY I: Establishing Graduate Courses in the United States *(continued)*

> people are available to direct, instruct, and supervise these programs. The need for knowledge of psychiatric nursing has been so generally recognised that requests for student affiliations in all areas of the country are far in excess of the courses and nurse instructors available. (Fitzsimmons, 1944b, p. 1167)

Fitzsimmons worked with a number of nursing schools, the NLNE, and the U.S. Public Health Service during this period to help them work through the complex funding maze in order to obtain grants for postgraduate courses in psychiatric nursing (NLNE, 1945). At the same time, with the end of World War II, the passing of the GI Bill offered nurses returning from war the option of further study with tuition costs covered. The National Mental Health Act, passed in 1946, and the establishment of the NIMH in 1948 with its extensive grant program, meant that large amounts of funds became available to universities looking to develop graduate education courses. One nurse who availed herself of both of these opportunities was Hildegard Peplau.

Hildegard Peplau and Interpersonal Relations in Nursing

Hildegard Peplau was born in 1909 in rural Pennsylvania to German immigrant parents. Like many young women of her age and time, she undertook nurses training because it was the most easily accessible education and occupational opportunity and meant she could stay close to home. Peplau undertook her initial training at Pottstown Hospital in Reading, Pennsylvania, and there she was introduced to psychiatric nursing by Arthur Noyes, the Chief Psychiatrist at Norristown State Hospital. Noyes had written texts, such as *A Textbook on Psychiatry for Students and Graduates in Schools of Nursing* (1927) and *Modern Clinical Psychiatry* (1934), and was president of the APA from

(continued)

CASE STUDY I: Establishing Graduate Courses in the United States *(continued)*

1954 to 1955. It was not, however, until much later that Peplau formally pursued her interest in psychiatric nursing. In the early 1940s, after working in a variety of nursing positions in New York City, Peplau first undertook a bachelor's degree in interpersonal psychology at Bennington College in Vermont, where she was also working as the college nurse. At Bennington, Peplau was exposed to the latest thinking in psychiatry, psychology, social psychiatry, and social work. By the 1940s, the college was home to some of the most influential names in psychology and psychiatry, with luminaries such as Erich Fromm, Frieda Fromm-Reichmann, and Harry Stack Sullivan all contributing to the program, with its strong focus on social psychiatry in the period leading up to World War II. In 1943, Peplau finished her degree and enrolled in the U.S. Army Nurse Corps. She was eventually posted to the U.S. Army's 312th Neuropsychiatric Field Hospital in the south of England. She found Army nursing frustrating, and psychiatric practice ad hoc and often unethical, struggling with the reliance on experimental and drug-dependent treatments and the lack of theoretical rigor. Personally and professionally she chafed under the Army's masculine hierarchy and the lack of respect accorded to her own expertise as a psychiatric specialist. Yet she was eventually given control of one whole ward, where she could bring her expertise into practice. She instituted a therapeutic program based on one-on-one interviews, group therapy, and occupational therapy (Callaway, 2002; Peplau, 1944).

In all of this work, Peplau saw the importance of the role of psychiatric and psychological theory, the need for practice based on research and evidence, and the unique opportunity for nurses to make a clear contribution to the therapeutic process. She knew, however, that the only reason she had been able to fight back against Army processes was because she had a thorough grounding in the knowledge, theory, and language of contemporary psychology and psychiatry. Her firm belief was that without

(continued)

CASE STUDY I: Establishing Graduate Courses in the United States *(continued)*

graduate courses aimed at teaching emerging nurses and future nurse educators these principles—indeed, without courses that were devoted to the specific practice of psychiatric nursing as an advanced specialty—the discipline itself would founder. To this end, when she returned from World War II in 1945, she enrolled in a graduate nurse education program at Teachers College (TC), Columbia University, where she also completed a PhD. In 1948 she was then employed at TC to begin the process of remodeling a graduate psychiatric nursing program, and solidified her position in the field of psychiatric nursing with the publication in 1952 of *Interpersonal Relations in Nursing: A Conceptual Frame of Reference for Psychodynamic Nursing* (Peplau, 1952). This groundbreaking book appeared in the same year that the APA published the first *Diagnostic and Statistical Manual* (*DSM-I*).

Yet her work was controversial and confronting, as it argued that nurses themselves could and should be therapists, acting autonomously from the psychiatrist. This would only be possible, however, if psychiatric nurses were fully versed in the latest theories and methods. When Peplau was hired to set up the brand new graduate psychiatric nursing program at Rutgers University in New Jersey, she was given carte blanche to do it her way in the absence of any existing standards. This was a time for experimentation—the NIMH was interested in any and all approaches to mental health, especially those that focused on therapy, recovery, and prevention. Peplau's colleague, Dorothy Mereness, noted the varying effects this had on the development of curricula: "Different places were developing different ideas. . . . We all got similar amounts of money, and all had to beat the bushes for their first class" (Mereness, 1985).

The essence of Peplau's program at Rutgers was psychotherapy. Students themselves underwent analysis (as Peplau herself had done) at the William Alanson White Institute in New York City (where Peplau was also a certified psychotherapist). This self-development was combined with theory and

(continued)

CASE STUDY I: Establishing Graduate Courses in the United States *(continued)*

clinical case studies. She was able to arrange placements for students at Greystone Psychiatric Hospital and students spent intensive time with a patient talking and recording observations. This was a practice that Peplau had learned from Frieda Fromm-Reichmann, entrusting that listening to even the most delusional and schizophrenic of patients could reveal meaning and symbols in their "word salad." She called this kind of training 1:1 relationship studies. But really, she explained, they "were moving in the direction of psychotherapy . . . we didn't call it that, we called it 1:1 and we called it talking with patients, and then we called it counseling and then we called it therapy. That took from 1948 until 1960" (Peplau, 1985).

"Talking with patients" was the essence of Peplau's therapeutic approach. She set out in *Interpersonal Relations in Nursing*, her subsequent text *Basic Principles of Patient Counseling* (1964), and many other articles (Peplau, 1960, 1962, 1963, 1964), the techniques and strategies for nurse-directed therapy that were part of comprehensive patient care. This method "requires a marked shift in emphasis from telling a patient how to behave in line with preconceived goals of the nurse, toward helping the patient to inquire and to find out what is going on with him" (Peplau, 1956, p. 191). It also required the active presence of the nurse, for the nurse to know his or her own values and anxieties, to put aside judgments and the need to control, and to learn to listen. This way of working was in direct contrast to the paternalism inherent to existing theories of care, which saw the nurses' role as "to do for" the patient what they were unable to do for themselves. Shifting the focus to the patient required the nurse to resist the urge to fix and control, and demanded instead that the nurse facilitate the patient's own experience. This was a major refocusing of the goal of nursing practice, and was made possible through the framework of psychodynamic nursing.

(continued)

CASE STUDY I: Establishing Graduate Courses in the United States *(continued)*

Peplau's theory of "interpersonal nursing" went on to have lasting and global impact, so that the concepts she developed—therapeutic use of self, thereness, talking with patients—have become so essential to disciplines beyond just psychiatric nursing that they are now taken for granted. Peplau herself was a hugely influential figure in professional nursing in the mid-20th century, not only running her own program, but also running seminars at other universities across the country, consulting to the NIHM, publishing, lecturing, and serving on numerous professional organizational boards, including on the NLNE's subcommittee on psychiatric nursing. From 1969 to 1974, she served as executive director, president, and second vice president of the American Nurses Association (Figure 6.2).

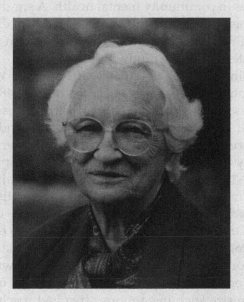

FIGURE 6.2 Dr. Hildegard Peplau, president, American Nurses Association 1970–1972.

Photo used with permission from American Nurses Association and the Howard Gottlieb Archival Research Center, Boston University.

POLICY SHIFTS IN THE 1960s AND 1970s

Peplau's biographer, Barbara Calloway (2002), has called Peplau "the psychiatric nurse of the century" and many may argue that her influence was wider even than this. However, the originality of Peplau's ideas was overshadowed in the later decades of the century with the move to biomedical approaches to psychiatric illness. Developments in the 1960s and 1970s shifted mental health policy. Peplau's model was predicated on the nurse having intense periods of time with patients, which was largely possible only in inpatient institutions. New professions such as social work and occupational therapy entered psychiatric care and teamwork emerged as a multidisciplinary approach to practice with stronger emphasis on rehabilitation and short-term treatment (Boschma, Yonge, & Mychajlunow, 2005). The advent of psychotropic medications in the 1950s as well as introduction of public health insurance programs during the 1960s further shifted policy. With the passing of the Community Mental Health Act of 1968, the disintegration of the institutional inpatient system began, resulting in new roles for nurses in community mental health. A similar shift occurred in Canadian mental health. In the next case study, we examine the emergence of such new roles for nurses, drawing from examples in the Canadian context (see Case Study II).

Public opinion about psychiatry after World War II had been shaped by popular movies, such as *The Snake Pit* (1948), which had had the effect of associating institutional care with stories of terrible conditions in archaic institutions, presided over by ill-minded psychiatrists, with little concern for patient welfare. In most Western countries, public controversy over poor conditions of mental hospitals grew stronger during the 1960s and 1970s, fueled by protest against authoritarian cultural and medical models, rising civic and patient rights movements, antipsychiatric critique, and a stronger voice of patients themselves (Goffman, 1961; Kesey, 1962). Canada was no exception (Moran & Wright, 2006). Large mental hospitals, for long the dominant, if not only, option for treatment, were now closed or downsized, although the timeline for such changes varied among states or provinces. The unmanageable size such institutions often had reached and a lack of patient rights stirred a public outcry among politicians and professionals as well as patients, a critique epitomized in the public mind through the film *One Flew Over the Cuckoo's Nest* (1975), based on Kesey's 1962 book by the same name.

Patient activism grew as well. In Canada, one of the first patient-led activist organizations, the Mental Patients' Association (MPA), was founded in Vancouver, British Columbia, in 1971; and in the United States, Judy Chamberlain became an influential spokesperson for mental health patients' rights (Chamberlain, 1978). As a result of these pressures, as well as the apparently mood-stabilizing effects of new psychotropic drugs and growing concerns over the cost of running large-scale institutions, mental health policy shifted toward deinstitutionalization of long-term hospitalized patients and new community-based services. For nurses, this shift had significant implications. As large numbers of discharged patients had to transition to living into the community, many nurses obtained new roles in community mental health, requiring new approaches to practice (Boschma, 2012; Church, 1987). An example of this process is explored in the next section.

CASE STUDY II: New Nursing Roles in Community Mental Health: A Canadian Example

In the construction of new community services, nurses had an essential but as yet ill-defined role and needed to carve out a new professional identity and approaches to practice that expanded their independence, therapeutic role, and capacity for leadership. New institutional structures, such as new psychiatric departments in general hospitals and new community-based mental health centers and outreach teams, formed the context of new nursing role development. Stories of community mental health nurses, shared in an oral history interview project conducted with mental health nurses in western Canada, provide insight into the way nurses transformed former institutional approaches into new rehabilitative practices and community outreach (Boschma, 2012, 2015; Boschma, Scaia, Bonifacio & Roberts, 2008). Drawing from these latter works, in this case study we specifically focus on the establishment of outpatient services in a new psychiatric department at the Foothills Provincial General Hospital in Calgary, Alberta, established around 1970.

(continued)

CASE STUDY II: New Nursing Roles in Community Mental Health: A Canadian Example *(continued)*

The story of Margaret Mandryk sheds light on the experience of these changes toward community mental health (Mandryk, 1999). Mandryk started her nursing career at Alberta (Mental) Hospital in Edmonton in 1962 at age 18. More than 30 years later, Mandryk remembered the many complex aspects of her work, which demonstrated that her career path was dramatically affected by the move toward community care. As she took on a new position in Calgary, her professional identity changed. She remembered how she became Calgary's first community mental health nurse, a new identity she actively began to embrace in 1966. At that time, she was most likely called a psychiatric nurse. Only in retrospect did she use the phrase "community mental health nurse," as it was in retrospect that she related to a transforming identity, a shifting context, for which the seeds were already planted in the third and last year of her training: "Even by my third year [in the mental hospital] things were a lot different in what we were studying, . . . looking at more things like the social factors of life, things like alcoholism" (Mandryk, 1999). Teaching moved away from the straight focus on anatomy and medications of the first year, she remembered.

Another formative influence during her training was a taste of community work she had been able to get. By the mid-1960s, the Alberta Hospitals both in Edmonton and Ponoka had begun to downsize and discharge their chronic mentally ill population:

> I did some community, a little bit of work with a social worker there at Alberta Hospital in Edmonton as part of my, um, I think it was an elective, . . . really enjoyed community work and often thought "Gee, that would be what I [would like to] do when I graduate," but again, you just, you just sort of dream about those sort of things, and when I came to Calgary I

(continued)

**CASE STUDY II: New Nursing Roles in Community Mental Health:
A Canadian Example** *(continued)*

started to look for work, there wasn't a whole lot open
for psychiatric nurses. (Mandryk, 1999)

Inspired by those experiences, however, Mandryk preferred to stay in psychiatry. What she dreamed of was indeed
not readily available because Calgary did not have a large
mental hospital, so jobs for psychiatric nurses were scarce. At
the same time, Alberta Hospital Ponoka (AH-Ponoka), a large
mental institution in the middle of the Canadian province of
Alberta, was discharging patents to the city of Calgary. This
required the development of the so-called "after-care services"
for patients discharged from AH-Ponoka. "After-care" refers
to the care patients need to make the transition after discharge
from the mental hospital. Such care, however, did not exist at
this time and had to be invented and made to work. These new
services needed nurses such as Mandryk, who actually understood these clients and the medications they were on, which
now needed monitoring, if not administering, in the community. Mandryk's experience was valued: "And so I went
to AH-Ponoka, I think the next Tuesday, . . . we traveled to
AH-Ponoka every Tuesday [to coordinate discharges] and we
went to AH-Ponoka the next Tuesday and they hired me and
that's how I had my job" (Mandryk, 1999). A new era of community mental health nursing began for Mandryk. She would take
on a key role in constructing and shaping it, as nurses trod new
ground in the grassroots development of skills and services in
the community. She developed new group work for discharged
patients in the community and helped develop community outreach when a new department of psychiatry was formed in
the Foothills Provincial General Hospital in the late 1960s. In her
story, we can trace the larger social changes of which she was part.

Joyce Taylor (pseudonym) was another nurse active at this
time of change (Taylor, 2004). Her strongest memories were of
patients: the people who had to make the transition from

(continued)

**CASE STUDY II: New Nursing Roles in Community Mental Health:
A Canadian Example** *(continued)*

institution to community, often at an older age, after having
spent years, if not decades, in the institution. In her story, she
reconstructed leaving the institution as a challenge. Despite
the optimism with which community care was developed,
many of the former patients ended up quite isolated once
again, and not all received the support they needed, Taylor
explained. Her stories about her clients illustrated how the formerly hospitalized patients were still not well when they
moved into the community, and they were not always able to
get the support they needed. Her account also gives unique
insight into the meaning of self-help in community care. In the
more unpredictable context of the community, support was a
complex process, not only to create or provide, but also to get.
Patients were visible only when they connected to a clinic or
agency on a regular basis, but there was no guarantee this
would actually happen. Taylor followed patients who came to
the Foothills Provincial General Hospital's psychiatric clinic in
Calgary on a monthly or biweekly basis. The psychiatrist leading
the follow-up program ran a group for schizophrenic patients.
During their visit, the patients attended the group, saw the
psychiatrist individually if necessary, and also saw the nurse.

Taylor worked primarily with elderly individuals who
were in their 70s at the time of their discharge from AH-Ponoka:
"They were becoming elderly because, you know, they'd been
in AH-Ponoka for so many years" (Taylor, 2004). Sometimes,
reinstitutionalization (in nursing homes or lodges) occurred as
these elderly clients became too frail. One frail elderly lady
Taylor (2004) visited in the community on a regular basis "was
somebody, you know, that survived, just barely survived, so
when she became extremely frail we were actually able to get
in the geriatric mental health team and they moved her to a
nursing home to spend her last days." Taylor (2004) continued
to point out that getting people with a psychiatric diagnosis
into a nursing home was very difficult at the time, but also

(continued)

**CASE STUDY II: New Nursing Roles in Community Mental Health:
A Canadian Example *(continued)***

essential: "I was having to move a lot of these people into nursing homes because they just were not surviving on their own
and there wasn't family support." Taylor observed how people
were functioning during home visits, and she tried to revitalize
connections with siblings, or sometimes with children of the
discharged person. Occasionally, she was able to find families,
but "they didn't understand, they weren't given the, the teaching about schizophrenia . . . and so this particular [elderly]
lady had a sister and a brother I was able to contact regarding
her care, but you had to do a fair amount of pushing to get, to
get the family involved" (Taylor, 2004).

For people living with mental illness in the community, a
"self-help" philosophy sometimes emerged out of necessity,
and peer help was a crucial survival strategy (Shimrat, 1997).
Emerging patterns of self-help have been looked upon both in
positive and negative terms, and are at the heart of the consumer movement that grew in the context of deinstitutionalization (Tomes, 2006). For some, these developments underscored
how psychiatry did not work, and that, as a result, consumers
or survivors had to rely on each other, in a context where actual
resources were lacking. Others saw self-help as the beginning
of a more independent life in the community, prompting healthy
coping mechanisms that helped people with mental illness
recover and survive (Tomes, 2006).

The stories of home visiting and community mental health
care demonstrate how the strategy to actively help people social-
ize, as well as the pressure former patients experienced to survive in a new context of "community," pushed a new agenda of
rehabilitation, in which people with mental illness took on an
active role in the management of their lives and care. Taylor's
and Mandryk's stories also illuminated how rehabilitation provided nurses the opportunity to construct a more independent,
therapeutically based professional identity. Finally, the stories
illustrate how the ideal of independence in the community was

(continued)

**CASE STUDY II: New Nursing Roles in Community Mental Health:
A Canadian Example** *(continued)*

fragile, difficult to achieve, and fraught with many new problems as the demand for community care increased and resources fell short. Many of the dilemmas and challenges of long-term institutional care were reproduced rather than resolved in the new community-based mental health services.

Establishing rehabilitation and community care in the 1960s and 1970s was a complex process constrained by pressures of funding and fragmentation (Fingard & Rutherford, 2011). From the stories, we learn that deinstitutionalization, increased reliance on psychiatric departments in general hospitals, and more community services have not resolved the complex problems people living with mental illness continue to face, including stigma, homelessness, disparities in access, and lack of specialized services (Kirby, 2005). The shift to community settings produced new, more fluid, and even more complex institutional contexts, raising the question whether we really can speak of a process of deinstitutionalization. As a result, persistent dilemmas of mental health care continue to be high on the health policy agenda—and nurses are called upon to make rehabilitative services work in an increasingly complex political and social context.

DISCUSSION AND CONCLUSION

Mental health sits at the intersection of a number of often-competing political and cultural philosophies about the nature and meaning of mental illness. Although there may be increased awareness and acceptance of the idea of mental illness, many in the community are unsure what this means, or how best to deal with the often complex and uncomfortable issues it can cause. Nurses need to be mediators of this process, negotiating the medical and scientific aspects of illness and treatments with the social and community expectations of care. Stigma about mental health is still strong, and can have devastating consequences for patients who are often severely marginalized by under-resourced services and the judgments of practitioners. People with mental illness from underserved communities are more likely to be incarcerated than treated medically, and are more vulnerable to violence and homelessness. Although the concept of social determinants of health is gaining increasing attention in general health care, more work needs to be done on understanding the link between environment and mental health, and more and better services continue to be needed as the rates of mental illness around the world continue to climb.

Nurses are at the frontline of mental health services in *all* aspects of health care, as deinstitutionalization has meant that there is no longer any real separation between mental and general health care. People with mental illness can and do present in all areas of nursing, and nurses must be able to recognize people's health challenges and act accordingly, with compassion and care, keeping patients' individual needs and rights balanced with potential risks to others. This raises many ethical dilemmas for nurses, who must act within the law but also seek to uphold human rights, increasingly difficult in a biomedical and risk-averse health care system. Somatic treatments and psychotropic drugs, while bringing benefits, can impinge on individuals' sense of autonomy and sovereignty over their own body, and nurses must recognize the position of power they hold over people in extremely vulnerable emotional states (Holmes & Gastaldo, 2002; Perron, Fluet, & Holmes, 2005).

Nurses in the past knew that this was a difficult and complex area of clinical practice, with wide-reaching social and cultural implications. Before psychiatric nursing emerged as an advanced practice or clinical specialty, nurses such as Laura Fitzsimmons and Hildegard Peplau identified the need for high-level, theoretically based, and clinically prepared psychiatric nurses, and set about creating the educational programs and professional associations that would ensure this level of practice. These nurses believed in the primacy of the nurse as a therapeutic agent and carved out a role for psychiatric nursing that encouraged independent practice, developing the core principles that continue to underpin not just psychiatric but also general nursing. By focusing on the patient and the concept of recovery, nursing itself became empowered as an interpersonal process, equipping nurses with the skills and knowledge they needed to imagine and create healthy, respectful, and compassionate relationships with patients (D'Antonio et al., 2014).

Nurses who experienced the subsequent shift from institutions to community-based services needed to invent practices and methods of care that had no precedent, and that could support people with a broad range of health, family, and social needs. They adapted the theory and practice of institutions to new circumstances, shifting the locus of care to communities, families, and peers. These nurses worked ever closer with patients themselves, learning and modeling valuable lessons about the importance of patients' rights and the imperative of person-centered care.

Despite continued advances in neuroscience and brain biology, mental health nursing is still essentially an interpersonal process. This is a unique and significant contribution of nurses to provide holistic care that seeks to combine mind, body, and spirit, thus facilitating a patient-driven approach to recovery. This is an increasingly difficult task as funds continue to be cut at the same time as rates of illness continue to rise. Nurses working in mental health today need ever more complex theoretical and interpersonal skills with which to negotiate the nexus between body and mind, between patients and families, and between families and communities. Nurses work across the spectrum in mental health, from homelessness to maternity, to youth and child health, to suicide prevention, and to public health. This is an exciting and challenging field, which psychiatric nurses in the past faced with critique, courage, and innovation, taking the reins of leadership to ensure that nurses themselves imagined and created their own knowledge, practice, and identity. In an increasingly biomedical model of health service provision, the imperative for nursing to stay cognizant of and critical about its unique role is more necessary than ever.

ACTIVITIES FOR TEACHING AND LEARNING

1. Watch the movie *The Snake Pit* from 1948.
   Reflect on the role of the nurses: Which different therapeutic techniques, effective or less effective, do you recognize? Reflect on the role of gender and power: How do these social forces shape the nurse–client relationship?
2. Watch the documentary on the Mental Patients' Association (MPA): "The inmates are running the asylum: Stories from the MPA" is a documentary about the group that transformed Canada's psychiatric landscape (DVD, 36-minutes; created by the MPA founders'

collective. © History of Madness Productions 2013; see, www.his
toryofmadness.ca/the-inmates-are-running-the-asylum).
3. Do patient and professional points of view about supportive communities for people with living with mental illness differ? How
effective was the model of peer help that the MPA developed? Would
it provide a model for service today?
4. Locate a copy of Peplau's book *Interpersonal Relations in Nursing* from
1952. What concepts, theories, and ideas do you recognize as fundamental to your own practice today?

REFERENCES

Borsay, A., & Dale, P. (Eds.). (2015). *Mental health nursing: The working lives of paid
carers in the nineteenth and twentieth centuries.* Manchester, England:
Manchester University Press.

Boschma, G. (2003). *The rise of mental health nursing: A history of psychiatric
care in Dutch Asylums 1890–1920.* Amsterdam, Netherlands: Amsterdam
University Press.

Boschma, G. (2012). Community mental health nursing in Alberta, Canada:
An oral history. *Nursing History Review, 20,* 103–135.

Boschma, G. (2013). Community mental health post-1950: Reconsidering nurses'
and consumers' identities. In P. D'Antonio, J. Fairman, & J. Whelan (Eds.),
Routledge handbook on the global history of nursing (pp. 237–258). London,
England: Routledge Taylor & Francis Group.

Boschma, G. (2015). Conducting oral history research in community mental
health nursing. In M. de Chesnay (Series Ed.), *Nursing research using historical methods: Qualitative research designs and methods in nursing* (pp. 85–104).
New York, NY: Springer Publishing.

Boschma, G., Scaia, M., Bonifacio, N., & Roberts, E. (2008). Oral history
research. In S. B. Lewenson & E. Krohn-Herrmann (Eds.), *Capturing nursing history: A guide to historical methods in research* (pp. 79–98). New York,
NY: Springer Publishing.

Boschma, G., Yonge, O., & Mychajlunow, L. (2005). Gender and professional
identity in psychiatric nursing practice in Alberta, Canada, 1930–1975.
Nursing Inquiry, 12(4), 243–255.

Callaway, B. J. (2002). *Hildegard Peplau: Psychiatric nurse of the century.* New
York, NY: Springer Publishing.

Chamberlain, J. (1978). *On our own: Patient-controlled alternatives to the mental health system*. New York, NY: Hawthorne Books.

Church, O. (1987). From custody to community in psychiatric nursing. *Nursing Research, 36*(1), 48–55.

D'Antonio, P. (2004). Relationships, reality and reciprocity with therapeutic environments: An historical case study. *Archives of Psychiatric Nursing, 18*(1), 11–16.

D'Antonio, P. (2006). *Founding friends: Families, staff, and patients at the Friends Asylum in early nineteenth-century Philadelphia*. Bethlehem, PA: Lehigh University Press.

D'Antonio, P., Beeber, L., Sills, G., & Nagle, M. (2014). The future in the past: Hildegaard Peplau and interpersonal relations in nursing. *Nursing Inquiry, 21*(4), 311–317.

Desjarlais, R., Eisenberg, L., Good, B., & Kleinman, A. (Eds.). (1995). *World mental health: Problems and priorities in low-income countries*. New York, NY: Oxford University Press.

Deutsch, A. (1937). *The mentally ill in America: A history of their care and treatment since colonial times*. New York, NY: Columbia University Press.

Deutsch, A. (1959). *The story of GAP*. New York, NY: Group for the Advancement of Psychiatry.

Dowbiggin, I. R. (1997). *Keeping America sane: Psychiatry and eugenics in the United States and Canada 1880–1940*. Ithaca, NY: Cornell University Press.

Fingard, J., & Rutherford, J. (2011). Deinstitutionalization and vocational rehabilitation for mental health consumers in Nova Scotia since the 1950s. *Histoire Sociale/Social History, 44*(88), 385–408.

Fitzpatrick, C. (1941). Letter to Allan Gregg (Rockefeller Foundation RG 1: Series 200, Box 70, Folder 850, American Psychiatric Association—Nursing 1941–1942), Rockefeller Archive Center, Sleepy Hollow, NY.

Fitzsimmons, L. (1944a). Report to Committee on Psychiatric Nursing, American Psychiatric Association (Rockefeller Foundation RG 1: Series 200, Box 71, Folder 852, American Psychiatric Association—Nursing 1944–1946), Rockefeller Archive Center, Sleepy Hollow, NY.

Fitzsimmons, L. (1944b). University-controlled advanced clinical programs in psychiatric nursing. *American Journal of Nursing, 44*(12), 1166–1169.

Goffman, E. (1961). *Asylums: Essays on the social situation of mental patients and other inmates*. New York, NY: Doubleday.

Gregg, A. (1945, July 18). [Note from Diary]. Rockefeller Foundation. Record Group 1.1. Series 200. United States (Medical Science) Box 71, Folder 852: American Psychiatric Association. Rockefeller Archive Center, Sleepy Hollow, NY.

Grinker, R. R., & Speigel, J. P., (1945). *Men under stress*. Philadelphia, PA: Blakiston.

Grob, G. (1991). *From asylum to community: Mental health policy in modern America*. Princeton, NJ: Princeton University Press.

Grob, G. (1994). *The mad among us: A history of the care of America's mentally ill*. New York, NY: The Free Press.

Hale, N. (1995). *Freud and the Americans*. Oxford, England: Oxford University Press.

Holmes, D., & Gastaldo, D. (2002). Nursing as means of governmentality. *Journal of Advanced Nursing, 38*(6), 557–565.

International Council of Nurses. (2008). Position statement on mental health. Geneva, Switzerland: International Council of Nurses (www.icn.ch).

Kesey, K. (1962). *One flew over the cuckoo's nest*. New York, NY: Viking Press.

Kirby, M. J. L. (2005). Mental health reform for Canada in the 21st century: Getting there from here. *Canadian Public Policy: Analyse de Politique, 31*(s1), 5–12.

Lieberman, J. A. (2015). *Shrinks: The untold story of psychiatry*. New York, NY: Little, Brown.

Litvak, A. (Director and Co-Producer). (1948). *The snake pit* [Motion picture]. United States: Twentieth Century-Fox.

Mandryk, M. (1999). *Oral history*. Oral History Collection, Museum and Archives, College and Association of Registered Nurses of Alberta, Edmonton, AB, Canada.

Menninger, W. C. (1948). *Psychiatry in a troubled world*. New York, NY: Macmillan.

Mereness, D. (1985). *Oral history*. Dorothy A. Mereness Papers, Barbara Bates Center for the Study of the History of Nursing, University of Pennsylvania School of Nursing, Philadelphia, PA.

Moran, J. E., & Wright, D. (Eds.). (2006). *Mental health and Canadian society: Historical perspectives*. Montreal, QC/Kingston, NY: McGill-Queen's University Press.

National League of Nursing Education (NLNE). (1945). *Courses in clinical nursing for graduate nurses: An advanced course in psychiatric nursing*. Prepared by

Subcommittee on Psychiatric Nursing of the Special Committee on Postgraduate Clinical Nursing Courses. New York, NY: National League of Nursing Education.

Olson, T. (1996). Fundamental and special: The dilemma of psychiatric-mental health nursing. *Archives of Psychiatric Nursing, 10*(1), 3–10.

Peplau, H. (1944, July). *Hildegard E. Peplau letters to sister Bertha Peplau.* Hildegard E. Peplau Papers, Schlesinger Library Collection, Radcliffe Institute for the Study of American Women, Harvard University, Cambridge, MA.

Peplau, H. (1952). *Interpersonal relations in nursing: A conceptual frame of reference for psychodynamic nursing.* New York, NY: Putnam.

Peplau, H. (1956). Present day trends in psychiatric nursing. *Neuropsychiatry, 3,* 190–204.

Peplau, H. (1960). Talking with patients. *American Journal of Nursing, 60*(7), 964–966.

Peplau, H. (1962). Interpersonal techniques: The crux of psychiatric nursing. *American Journal of Nursing, 62*(6), 50–54.

Peplau, H. E. (1963). Interpersonal relations and the process of adaptation. *Nursing Science, 1*(4), 272–279.

Peplau, H. (1964). *Basic principles of patient counseling.* Philadelphia, PA: Smith, Kline & French.

Peplau, H. (1985). *Oral history.* Hildegard E. Peplau Papers, Barbara Bates Center for the Study of the History of Nursing, University of Pennsylvania School of Nursing, Philadelphia, PA.

Perron, A., Fluet, C., & Holmes, D. (2005). Agents of care and agents of the state: Bio-power and nursing practice. *Journal of Advanced Nursing, 50*(5), 536–544.

Pressman, J. (1998). *Last resort: Psychosurgery and the limits of medicine.* New York, NY: Columbia University Press.

Rees, J. R. (1945). *The shaping of psychiatry by war.* London, England: W. W. Norton.

Saxena, S., & Barrett, T. (2007). *Nurses in mental health: Atlas 2007.* Geneva, Switzerland: World Health Organization and International Council of Nurses.

Shimrat, I. (1997). *Call me crazy: Stories from the Mad Movement.* Vancouver, BC, Canada: Press Gang.

Taylor, J. (pseudonym). (2004). *Oral history.* Interview by A. Lane, conducted as part of a study on the transformation of mental health care in Alberta, 1905–1975. [Tape recording and transcript held at UBC by PI G. Boschma].

Tomes, N. (2006). The patient as a policy factor: A historical case study of the Consumer/Survivor Movement in mental health. *Health Affairs, 25,* 720–729.

United Nations General Assembly. (1991). Principles for the protection of persons with mental illness and for the improvement of mental health care. Retrieved from http://www.un.org/documents/ga/res/46/a46r119.htm

World Health Organization. (1946). Preamble to the Constitution of the World Health Organization as adopted by the International Health Conference, New York, 19–22 June, 1946; signed on 22 July 1946 by the representatives of 61 States (Official Records of the World Health Organization, no. 2, p. 100) and entered into force on 7 April 1948. Retrieved from http://www.who .int/about/definition/en/print.html

World Health Organization. (2002). *Nations for mental health: Final report* [WHO/ NMH/MSD/MPS/02.02]. Geneva, Switzerland: Author.

Chapter 7: Educational Pathways for Differentiated Nursing Practice: A Continuing Dilemma

APRIL D. MATTHIAS

Refusal to state frankly a clear differentiation of levels of nursing constitutes one of the most significant problems facing nurses today.
(Rogers, 1961, p. 4)

The nursing profession is moving forward with a renewed focus to advance the education of the RN and define the bachelor of science in nursing (BSN) degree as the minimum educational preparation for professional nursing practice. Today's renewed focus is due, in part, to research published in the past 14 years demonstrating improved patient outcomes when the nursing workforce includes a high percentage of BSN-prepared nurses (Aiken, Clarke, Cheung, Sloane, & Silber, 2003; Aiken, Clarke, Sloane, Sochalski, & Silber, 2002; Blegen et al., 2013; Kutney-Lee, Sloane, & Aiken, 2013). Despite efforts to increase the percentage of BSN-prepared nurses, different educational pathways continue to produce nurses and these nurses legally share the same nursing practice role based on licensure. Different educational pathways leading to the same licensure exam have challenged efforts to specify an entry-level RN's professional identity and practice role based on education. Differentiation would mean that a nurse's role on the unit or in the community would vary based on educational level of skills and knowledge. Someone with a bachelor's degree in nursing would stand out from someone with a diploma or an associate degree. When we cannot distinguish between and among the varying levels, it confuses both the public and the profession. Who is a "registered" nurse and how does the educational preparation influence the nurse's role? This chapter examines how education shapes the role of the nurse and explores the issues related to the enduring confusion about education, practice, and roles. It does so by examining the historical development of three educational pathways into nursing and the unintended consequences of each as we continue to treat them all the same.

Historical analysis of the three prevalent educational pathways to entry-level RN practice—the diploma, BSN, and associate degree in nursing (ADN) programs—demonstrates that each pathway was developed with the intent to advance the education of the nurse and differentiate, based on education, a specific professional identity and practice role for the nurse (Matthias, 2011). The pathway developments succeeded in advancing the education of some nurses, yet did not accomplish the intended differentiation. The historical persistence of the multiple educational pathways must be considered as the profession moves forward in efforts to advance the education of today's nurses.

This chapter presents the histories of early programs of the three educational pathways: the Bellevue School of Nursing (1873), as the diploma case study; the University of Cincinnati (UC) School of Nursing and Health (1916), as the BSN case study; and the Cooperative Research Project (CRP) in Junior and Community College Education for Nursing (1952), as the ADN case study. An informed historical perspective can help nurse leaders determine the viability of the renewed focus and effectiveness of current efforts to advance the education of the nurse requiring the bachelor's degree in nursing as the minimal requirement for entry into practice.

BACKGROUND

Pleas to Differentiate Practice Based on Education

Early- to mid-20th century reports on nursing education revealed deficiencies in nursing education, specifically the hospital-based training programs, and also recognized the need to differentiate nursing practice by the educational preparation of the nurse (Brown, 1948; Committee on the Grading of Nursing Schools, 1934; Goldmark, 1923). The addition of the ADN pathway in 1952 as the third pathway to RN practice ignited a volatile debate in nursing. The literature in the 1960s and 1970s exploded with nurse leaders' pleas for differentiation of nursing practice roles among the diploma, ADN, and BSN RNs. Noted nurse theorist, Martha Rogers, defined lack of differentiated nursing practice by educational preparation as "monuments of conflict and confusion" and labeled the refusal to differentiate nursing practice as "one of the most significant problems facing nurses" (Rogers, 1961, p. 4). In 1965, the American Nurses Association (ANA) and the National League for Nursing (NLN) both issued position papers that encouraged differentiated practice and classification of the nursing roles as technical and professional. They also called for the delineation of the educational programs to prepare each role or the call to action to do so. Due to a strong opposition from the nurse leaders of diploma and ADN programs and the diploma and ADN-prepared nurses themselves who would assume the title "technical," neither organization maintained its position. In 1978, the ANA once again published a position paper very similar to the 1965 paper proposing differentiated practice but this time put a timeline on the resolutions proposed. The resolutions did not meet the proposed deadlines. By 1982, both the ANA and NLN shared official agreement that the BSN should be minimal preparation for "professional" nursing practice and the NLN "supported all education programs in nursing, in response, . . . to the social reality" (Haase, 1990, p. 124).

Numerous studies between 1990 and 1999 concerned differentiation of entry-level RN practice. All the studies reported positive and beneficial outcomes, such as increased patient satisfaction, efficient and effective utilization of scarce nursing resources, empowered decision making, and preparation of graduates for a more specified role (Bellack & Loquist, 1999; Koerner, 1992; Malloch, Milton, & Jobes, 1990; Vena & Oldaker, 1994). Only two studies reported barriers to the implementation of differentiated practice, including the lack of appreciation and value for the "other" educationally prepared nurses, ignorance, the lack of current differentiated compensation, the insufficient supply of BSN nurses, and a decrease in the number of applicants to nursing programs (Bellack & Loquist, 1999; Pitts-Willhelm, Nicolai, & Koerner, 1991). Although beneficial evidence supporting differentiated practice existed in research, the implementation of differentiated practice between entry-level RNs remained minimal.

CASE STUDY I: The Diploma Pathway: Bellevue School of Nursing

The advancement of medicine and medical education along with the development of public hospitals called for a new nurse role within the public sphere. Florence Nightingale successfully molded the role of the middle-class trained nurse to encompass womanly attributes and intelligence into a subordinate and distinct, gender-specific role from that of the physician. Nightingale's success in healing the sick and injured soldiers during the Crimean War gained worldwide attention. Her philosophy of the trained nurse and the model of her training school, the Nightingale Home and Training School for Nurses at St. Thomas' Hospital in England, served to design the American trained nurse.

The New York State Charities Aid Association founded and led by Louisa Lee Schuyler set out on a mission to establish a Nightingale-model training school for nurses at the Bellevue Hospital to improve the care and conditions of the hospital (Giles, 1949, p. 67; Schuyler, 1912). Women within the association were assigned to investigate conditions of the hospital over several months to gather evidence for the training school proposal. It is important to note that prior to the opening of this school, typically anyone could call themselves a nurse, with or without training. Bellevue Hospital was staffed by untrained women who were often serving time as vagrants, paupers, or prisoners, many of whom could not read or write. Care at night was given by a night-watchman and it was his job to contact a physician if a patient became ill. Rats and vermin ran wild through the halls of the hospital, contributing to the unsafe and unsanitary conditions of a public hospital (Alumnae Association of Bellevue, Pension Fund Committee, 1915). With the assistance of physician Walker Gill Wylie, these women discovered and recorded deplorable conditions and care of patients (Giles, 1949). The proposal to open a training school originally received opposition from the Bellevue Hospital Medical Board. Many of the physicians opposed educating women to become nurses. Wylie agreed to travel to Europe to study the

(continued)

CASE STUDY I: The Diploma Pathway: Bellevue School of Nursing
(continued)

Nightingale model to "get the practical information" needed to alleviate the physicians' concerns (Giles, 1949, p. 83). Nightingale addressed Wylie in a letter outlining the standards of the Nightingale model (Nightingale, 1872). This letter guided the formation and continued operation of the school for many years. Within Nightingale's letter, she delineated the role of nursing from medicine and outlined the gender-specific subordinate role of the nurse to the physician. Nightingale further described a nurse's skill and competence to include the execution of medical directions through the art of cleanliness, ventilation, diet, and so forth, and the nurse's knowledge of the rationale for doing things a certain way. With this new knowledge, the Bellevue Medical Board (Figure 7.1) and, reluctantly, the Commissioners of Public Charities and Corrections accepted the proposal and provided six hospital wards for the training of nurses but with the strict condition of no additional cost to the hospital (Nutting & Dock, 1935, p. 383). Funds were secured, students were recruited, and a Nightingale-trained superintendent was hired for the training school to open on May 1, 1873.

By using the Nightingale-model, Bellevue established itself as a place to educate a secular trained nurse, focused on attracting women from the middle class. Bellvue's founders established a school that would "benefit not only Bellevue [in improving the care of the hospitalized patient], but all public hospitals, and also to train nurses for the sick in private homes and for the work among the poor" (Nutting & Dock, 1935, p. 384). Other schools like Bellevue opened around the same time (Figure 7.2).

Nightingale influenced training schools offered improved patient care in hospitals (Rosenberg, 1987). The apprenticeship model allowed hospitals to staff the wards with student nurses. As a result, hospitals benefitted economically from the use of this workforce. Students'

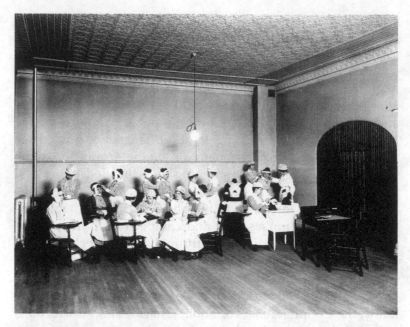

FIGURE 7.1 Bandaging class, Bellevue School of Nursing, ca. 1920.
Source: Bellevue

learning focused on the direct care of the patients rather than the educational experiences (Ashley, 1976; Reverby, 1987; Rosenberg, 1987). Upon graduation, the trained nurse was replaced by the next class of student nurses to provide the much needed patient care. Although some of the graduating nurses were hired as superintendants of the training school or as a teachers, most found work in private duty or in public health. During these early years, control of nursing roles and scope of practice rested in the hands of physicians, both in hospitals and in the realm of private duty nursing where the trained nurse and the untrained nurse both worked. This led to the trained nurse competing for private-duty nursing work with untrained nurses (Ashley, 1976; Reverby, 1987; Matthias, 2015).

The desire to professionalize nursing practice and differentiate a practice role for the trained nurse over the untrained nurse initiated efforts to standardize nurse training in the late 19th century. Nurse superintendents recognized the hospitals' paternalistic control over nursing education and practice, so they formed the American Society of Superintendents of Training Schools for Nurses in 1893 (later to

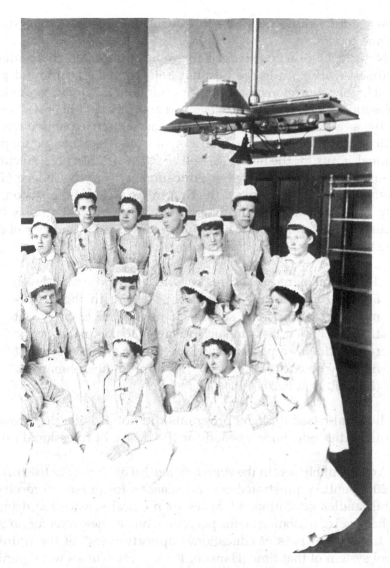

FIGURE 7.2 Bellevue School of Nursing class, 1893.
Source: Bellevue

become the National League of Nursing Education (NLNE) in 1912 and then the NLN in 1952). The major purpose of the Society was to "establish and maintain a universal standard of training" to regain control of nursing (Stewart, 1950, p. 150). Nurse leaders sought registration for nurses in order to control standardization of education and practice.

Nurse leaders acknowledged the rapidly changing environment of nurses' work both in the hospital and in public health and proposed higher education for nurses. As education for all the recognized professions in the United States evolved and included liberal studies, nursing as a developing profession also needed an expanded liberal studies education. Liberal education would also assist to secure professional status for the nurse. Russell (1959), assistant to the executive officer of the Institute of Higher Education at Teachers College (TC), Columbia University, prepared the first in the series of reports on the study of liberal education in undergraduate professional schools that concentrated on nursing. He explains the connection between liberal education and professional status in this way:

> The liberal ingredient brings knowledge to its humane level, and therefore forms an essential element in the performance of professional service. If nurses are to carry out their appointed tasks in such a way as to command public recognition as a profession in the fullest sense, they must not only be educated, but educated in the liberal manner. (Russell, 1959, p. 20)

The hospital-based diploma programs did not provide this broader liberal studies education needed for the desired professional nurse role.

Articles published in the *American Journal of Nursing* at the turn of the 20th century illustrated several reasons for nurses to receive a liberal studies education: advances in medical science requiring a "higher level of reasoning on the part of the nurse"; new roles for nurses; and the "narrowness of educational opportunities" of the training school system of that time (Hanson, 1988, p. 61). Nurses were gaining responsibility for advanced skills once performed by the physicians, and the physicians relied more on the nurses' assessment of physiological signs and symptoms. A broader education was necessary to enhance the nurse's ability to reason, think critically, and adapt, for no two patient situations were ever the same (Hanson, 1988).

CASE STUDY II: The BSN Pathway: University of Cincinnati (UC) School of Nursing and Health

In 1916 a dual diploma/BS degree program in nursing was established when the School of Nursing and Health of the Cincinnati General Hospital moved to a department within the UC College of Medicine at the University of Cincinnati (UC) (UC Board of Trustees, 1916). The training of nurses would provide a liberal course of studies in the undergraduate program that would be consistent with other professional programs offered at that time (UC Board of Trustees, 1915). The graduates of this new program would be equipped to provide hospital-based and private-duty nursing care, as well as receive the educational background that was needed for the public health role (Matthias, 2015).

It is historically important to note that the movement of nurse training to the university began in 1909 with the University of Minnesota (UM). The difference between the UM and the UC is that the UM training school fell under the university auspices; however, the curriculum of the training did not result in a bachelor's degree. Unlike the UC, the UM lacked a full liberal studies curriculum until 1919 (Powell, 1937).

Laura R. Logan newly hired as the superintendent of the School for Nursing and Health of the Cincinnati General Hospital on September 1, 1914, pressed forward with the vision of advancing the education of nurses and embracing the educational philosophy of university education (Officers, Boards, and Departments of the City of Cincinnati, 1914). Logan viewed the role of institutions that educate and train nurses to be "subserving [sic] not merely the immediate need of a hospital, but responsible for preparation of professional members of society, concerned . . . with the health and welfare of a community" (Logan, 1920, p. 15). Logan's desire to prepare graduates for a broader role beyond hospital nursing and for the role of the public health nurse grew evident in the changes she made.

Many changes to the curriculum resulted. Students earned credit hours for classroom and practice courses. Instruction

(continued)

CASE STUDY II: The BSN Pathway: University of Cincinnati (UC)
School of Nursing and Health *(continued)*

occurred in two parts: courses in the school of nursing consisting of 43 credit hours and practice courses in the wards, diet kitchen, and operating rooms consisting of 29 credit hours (Rosnagle & Darrington, 1950). As early as November 1914, Logan secured agreements from the UC College of Medicine professors, also responsible for the medical services in the hospital, to assist in the lectures and demonstrations in anatomy, physiology, bacteriology, pathology, pharmacology, and therapeutics (Officers, Boards, and Departments of the City of Cincinnati, 1914; Rosnagle & Darrington, 1950). In addition, Logan added a course in elementary sociology taught by a UC professor of the College of Liberal Arts on the university grounds (Logan, 1941). Lectures added to the nursing courses included Hygiene and Sanitation, Psychology, Hospital and Household Economy, and History of Nursing. Furthermore, electives available to the student nurses by 1915 included instruction and practice in Hospital Social Service, Modern Philanthropy, and Public Health Nursing (Rosnagle & Darrington, 1950). In 1914, Logan gained supervision of the nursing department within the tuberculosis (TB) sanatorium of the Cincinnati General Hospital with a forward intention to develop an optional course in TB nursing for the nursing school (Officers, Boards, and Departments of the City of Cincinnati, 1914). Logan expanded the curriculum of the training school to better coincide with a university, liberal studies curriculum and to better prepare the nurse for the expanding roles within the community.

Despite the forward vision of nurse leaders such as Logan, degree programs to prepare entry-level professional nurses did not rapidly develop. As late as 1951, less than 5% of the 102,509 students enrolled in nursing programs received their entire collegiate nursing education, both general and nursing courses, directly from the collegiate institution in which they were enrolled (Bridgman, 1953). Greater than 90% of nursing students received their entire nurse training in diploma hospital schools and the remaining students enrolled in collegiate institutions received the general education courses from the college and the nursing courses "in hospital schools with instruction by hospital school teachers in classes usually shared with diploma students" (Bridgman, 1953, p. 16). The latter programs, dual diploma/BS programs, proved to be a means of perpetuating the apprenticeship model rather than elevating the education of the nurse to a professional level because the nursing courses still remained within a hospital school (Bridgman, 1953). Hospital-based, diploma programs maintained a strong existence and produced the greater majority of nurses.

CASE STUDY III: The ADN Pathway: Cooperative Research Project (CRP)

In response to the mid-20th century drive to move nursing education into colleges and universities, and to the need created by the post–World War II nursing shortage, the 2-year community-based college program in nursing was developed. Starting in 1952, the ADN educational pathway was designed to advance the education of nurses as well as to differentiate technical and professional entry-level RN roles. Developed by Mildred Montag, a doctoral student and faculty member at TC, Columbia University in New York, the newly proposed ADN educational model was designed to differentiate nursing functions from those in other educational pathways. Montag developed a plan to establish a 2-year program in community colleges, then called junior colleges, graduating nurses with associate degrees in nursing. These new graduates would be educated in shools rather than in the hospitals, and thus, as Matthias (2015) noted, would be more educated than a diploma nurse from a hospital based program. The 2-year model was based on the education of the student rather than the apprentice model of the Nightingale schools, which treated students as workers rather than learners. Montag's work was in keeping with the long-held goal of nurse educators at the time to move the education of nurses out of the hospitals and into the American system of higher education. This ADN nurse took

(continued)

CASE STUDY III: The ADN Pathway: Cooperative Research Project (CRP) *(continued)*

the same licensing exam as all trained nurses but would enter as a technical nurse (Matthias, 2015; Montag, 1951). The technical nurse practice role was restricted to repetitive and routine situations in bedside care that required skilled techniques and exercise of judgment; thus, it was more limited in scope than the baccalaureate-educated professional nurse. Montag (1951) proposed that the technical nurse would provide nursing care under the supervision of a BSN-prepared RN. Montag's research provided the framework and the curriculum for the experimental programs of the CRP in Junior and Community College Education for Nursing (Matthias, 2015; "Research and Experimentation in Junior Colleges," 1951). Between 1952 and 1955, seven programs were established through the CRP. The success of the programs within the CRP was such that there was a rapid increase of this new and innovative model at community colleges across the country.

Montag's differentiated practice model included only the professional BSN RN, the technical ADN RN, and the nurse's aide. Montag's practice model did not identify a role for the diploma RN and therefore failed to differentiate nursing practice for all the differently prepared nurses who were practicing at the time. The research outcomes of the CRP led to the rapid growth of ADN programs within the community college system, and influenced a decrease, though not elimination, of diploma programs (Matthias, 2015). In spite of Montag's differentiation of roles in the education of ADN nurses, this differentiation was never clearly implemented in practice. The graduates all sat for the same licensure exams, regardless of educational levels. Hospitals thus defined the role and functions of the RN based on licensure and not educational preparation; and therefore, the practice of diploma, ADN, and BSN RNs was not differentiated (Advisory Committee on the Cooperative Research Project in Junior and Community College Education for Nursing, 1956).

DISCUSSION AND CONCLUSION

Despite efforts and evidence, the lack of practice differentiation based on the education of the entry-level RN continues today. Although there are minimal diploma programs today producing nurses, the diploma, ADN, and BSN program graduates remain eligible to obtain an RN license and practice under the same scope of practice with no differentiation based on education.

The research demonstrating improved patient outcomes with a high percentage of BSN nurses in the workforce has created a paradigm shift, and efforts are now aimed toward requiring a BSN for the entry-level professional nurse. State legislative proposals ("BSN in 10") requiring nurses to obtain a BSN degree within 10 years of initial licensure, and the Institute of Medicine's (IOM) *The Future of Nursing: Leading Change, Advancing Health* report recommendation ("80 by '20") calling for an increase in the proportion of BSN RNs to 80% by the year 2020, serve as examples of this shift (IOM, 2011; NJ Legislature Senate Bill S1258, 2012–2013; NY State Assembly Senate Bill S00628, 2013–2014). Both call for an increased percentage of BSN-prepared RNs in the nursing workforce but lack guidelines for differentiation of practice based on educational preparation of the nurse (Matthias, 2015). Throughout the United States, nurses with different entry-level educational preparations are eligible to be licensed and practice as RNs without differentiation based on education. Currently, more than 55% of RNs entering nursing practice do so without a BSN preparation (American Association of Colleges of Nursing [AACN], 2014; Budden et al., 2013).

The persistence of the multiple educational pathways cannot be ignored in light of the contemporary research demonstrating a correlation between the educational preparation of the nurse and improved patient outcomes. The evidence has the potential to differentiate a specific professional identity and practice role for the RN based on education in more than one way. The research could guide the profession to define the BSN for entry into RN practice and thus require closing the other pathways, or conversely, clearly differentiate RN practice based on education.

The cases studies illustrate that each educational pathway development served as an attempt to differentiate a specific practice role for the professional nurse based on educational preparation. In addition, the three educational pathways, although successful in advancing the education of some nurses, did not accomplish differentiated nursing practice. The continued use of differently prepared nurses in the same practice role challenged differentiation efforts. Today, a potential paradigm shift is noted as the outcome-based research has shifted employers' attention to the nurse's education and not just licensure (American Nurses Credentialing Center [ANCC], 2015; Trautman, 2015).

This history also reveals that nurses at times were fearful of losing their nurse identity or practice role and resisted efforts to advance the education of nurses, or differentiate practice or licensure based on education. A greater number of non-BSN nurses are returning to school to earn a BSN degree but largely due to employer preference and to ensure job security. Fear of needing to move away from a direct care practice role with an advanced education is still present for some nurses (Matthias & Kim-Godwin, 2016; Robert Wood Johnson Foundation [RWJF], 2013).

Over the years, strategies to advance the education of the nurse and differentiate a professional identity and practice role for the entry-level nurse lacked essential elements for success. Failure to clearly define a practice role with specific functions based on education allowed the unguided use of some nurses in each case study. As noted, the current "BSN in 10" legislative proposals and the "80 by '20" IOM recommendation also do not differentiate a practice role among the differently prepared RNs.

In addition, the lack of a phased plan for termination of other educational pathways allowed for the continued production of nurses from multiple program types. A phased plan to terminate remaining diploma and ADN programs is still lacking in current efforts. The "BSN in 10" proposals and the IOM report both support continuance of diploma and ADN programs to produce nurses, although the BSN degree is preferred. Transition programs do, however, exist to assist nurses in obtaining higher degrees (RWJF, 2013).

The scope of practice is based on RN licensure, not educational preparation of the RN. The literature shows that any change in licensure that would more accurately reflect differentiated practice roles for the diploma, ADN, and BSN RNs have proven to be both challenging and unrealistic to accomplish (Donley & Flaherty, 2002; Donley & Flaherty, 2008; Matthias, 2015; Nelson, 2002; Smith, 2009). The American Association of Colleges of Nurses (AACN) and the National League for Nursing (NLN) developed competencies for all entry-level RNs that rely on educational preparation to differentiate practice without the need to change state licensure requirements (AACN, 2008; NLN, 2010). Organizational clinical ladder models that include competencies that are based on the nurse's level of education can also be useful in continued attempts by health care institutions to differentiate the nurse's practice according to educational preparation (Matthias, 2015; Watts, 2010).

To ensure success of today's efforts to advance the education of nurses for improved patient outcomes, the identified barriers and flawed strategies need to be recognized and corrected. A broadened understanding of the past will assist nurse leaders to make evidence-based, informed decisions today. As the nursing profession moves forward to advance the education of nurses through policy changes, whether at the organizational level or state and national legislative level, success will be possible if the historical barriers are addressed and flawed strategies are considered. Whether the profession moves forward to require a BSN degree for entry into professional RN practice or to clearly differentiate RN practice based on the nurse's educational preparation, historical study is instrumental to guide contemporary policy regarding the education, professional identity, and practice role of the entry-level RNs. It is incumbent upon the reader to consider why the profession has argued about the differentiation of practice for decades without resolving the issue—even in the face of the evidence that shows better educated nurses provide better quality and safer care at the bedside.

ACTIVITIES FOR TEACHING AND LEARNING

1. How can the roles of different educationally prepared RNs be differentiated in your work setting?
2. Debate the pros and cons to phasing out diploma and ADN programs.
3. What other work-related factors/variables need to be taken into consideration to advance the education of the entry-level nurse to the baccalaureate degree?
4. Compare and contrast the existence and issues with the multiple entry-level educational pathways to the multiple doctoral pathways for nurses—EdD, DNSc, PhD, and now DNP.

5. Why do these three pathways still exist in the United States and not in other countries such as the United Kingdom, Australia, or Canada?

REFERENCES

Advisory Committee on the Cooperative Research Project in Junior and Community College Education for Nursing. (1956). *Report of fifth meeting of the Advisory Committee on the Cooperative Research Project in Junior and Community College Education for Nursing, January 16–17, 1956.* New York, NY: Teachers College, Columbia University. Archives of the Department of Nursing Education, Gottesman Library, Teachers College, Columbia University, New York, NY.

Aiken, L. H., Clarke, S. P., Cheung, R. B., Sloane, D., & Silber, J. (2003). Educational levels of hospital nurses and surgical patient mortality. *Journal of the American Medical Association, 290*(12), 1617–1623. doi:10.1001/jama.290.12.1617

Aiken, L. H., Clarke, S. P., Sloane, D. M., Sochalski, J., & Silber, J. (2002). Hospital nurse staffing and patient mortality, nurse burnout, and job dissatisfaction. *Journal of the American Medical Association, 288*(16), 1987–1993. doi:10.1001/jama.288.16.1987

Alumnae Association of Bellevue, Pension Fund Committee. (1915). *Bellevue: A short history of Bellevue Hospital and of the training schools.* New York, NY: Author. Retrieved from https://ia800300.us.archive.org/31/items/bellevueshorthis00grif/bellevueshorthis00grif_bw.pdf

American Association of Colleges of Nursing. (2008). *The essentials of baccalaureate education for professional nursing practice.* Washington, DC: Author. Retrieved from http://www.aacn.nche.edu/education-resources/BaccEssentials08.pdf

American Association of Colleges of Nursing. (2014, April). *Nursing shortage fact sheet.* Washington, DC: Author. Retrieved from http://www.aacn.nche.edu/media-relations/NrsgShortageFS.pdf

American Nurses Credentialing Center. (2015). Magnet® Recognition Program overview. Retrieved from http://www.nursecredentialing.org/Magnet/ProgramOverview.Aspx

Ashley, J. A. (1976). *Hospitals, paternalism, and the role of the nurse.* New York, NY: Teachers College Press.

Bellack, J. P., & Loquist, R. S. (1999). Employer responses to differentiated nursing education. *Journal of Nursing Administration, 29*(9), 4–8, 32. Retrieved from http://journals.lww.com/jonajournal/Citation/1999/09000/Employer_ Responses_to_Differentiated_Nursing.3.aspx

Blegen, M. A., Goode, C. J., Park, S. H., Vaughn, T., & Spetz, J. (2013). Baccalaureate education in nursing and patient outcomes. *Journal of Nursing Administration, 42*(2), 89–92. doi:10.1097/NNA.0b013e31827f2028

Bridgman, M. (1953). *Collegiate education for nurses.* New York, NY: Russell Sage Foundation.

Brown, E. L. (1948). *Nursing for the future: A report prepared for National Nursing Council.* New York, NY: Russell Sage Foundation.

Budden, J. S., Zhong, E. H., Moulton, P., & Cimiotti, J. P. (2013). Highlights of the National Workforce Survey of Registered Nurses. *Journal of Nursing Regulation, 4*(2), 5–14. doi:10.1016/S2155-8256%2815%2930151-4

Committee on the Grading of Nursing Schools. (1934). *Nursing schools today and tomorrow: Final report of the Committee on the Grading of Nursing Schools.* New York, NY: National League of Nursing Education.

Donley, R., & Flaherty, M. J. (2002). Revisiting the American Nurses Association's first position on education for nurses. *Online Journal of Issues in Nursing, 7*(2). Retrieved from http://www.nursingworld.org/MainMenuCategories/ANA Marketplace/ANAPeriodicals/OJIN/TableofContents/Volume72002/No2 May2002/RevisingPostiononEducation.html

Donley, R., & Flaherty, M. J. (2008). Revisiting the American Nurses Association's first position on education for nurses: A comparative analysis of the first and second position statements on the education for nurses. *Online Journal of Issues in Nursing, 13*(2). Retrieved from http://www.nursingworld.org/ MainMenuCategories/ANAMarketplace/ANAPeriodicals/OJIN/Tableof Contents/vol132008/No2May08/ArticlePreviousTopic/EntryIntoPractice Update.html

Giles, D. (1949). *A candle in her hand: A story of nursing schools at Bellevue Hospital.* New York, NY: G. P. Putnam's Sons.

Goldmark, J. (1923). *Nursing and nursing education in the United States.* New York, NY: MacMillan.

Haase, P. T. (1990). *The origins and rise of associate degree nursing education.* Durham, NC: Duke University Press.

Hanson, K. S. (1988). *A historical analysis of liberal education in nursing education, 1893–1952.* Ann Arbor, MI: University Microfilms International.

Institute of Medicine. (2011). *The future of nursing: Leading change, advancing health.* Washington, DC: National Academies Press. Retrieved from http://

www.nationalacademies.org/hmd/Reports/2010/The-Future-of
-Nursing-Leading-Change-Advancing-Health.aspx

Koerner, J. (1992). Differentiated practice: The evolution of professional nursing. *Journal of Professional Nursing, 8*(6), 335–341. doi:10.1016/8755-7223(92)
90096-H

Kutney-Lee, A., Sloane, D. M., & Aiken, L. H. (2013). An increase in the number of nurses with baccalaureate degrees is linked to lower rates of post-
surgery mortality. *Health Affairs, 32*(3), 579–586. doi:10.1377/hlthaff.2012.0504

Logan, L. (1920). Nursing in Cincinnati, 1820–1920. *University of Cincinnati
Medical Bulletin, 1*(1), 1–19.

Logan, L. (1941). *The place of the university in the nursing profession.* Unpublished
speech at the University of Cincinnati School of Nursing and Health
Graduation (Folder: Laura Logan). Archives of the Wedbush Centre,
College of Nursing, University of Cincinnati, Cincinnati, OH.

Malloch, K. M., Milton, D. A., & Jobes, M. O. (1990). A model for differentiated
nursing practice. *Journal of Nursing Administration, 20*(2), 20–26. Retrieved
from http://journals.lww.com/jonajournal/abstract/1990/02000/a_model_
for_differentiated_nursing_practice.7.aspx

Matthias, A. D. (2011). *Reframing disorder: Gender, class, and the history of the
resurfacing debate in nursing.* Ann Arbor, MI: University Microfilms
International. Retrieved from http://thescholarship.ecu.edu/handle/
10342/3672

Matthias, A. D. (2015). Making the case for differentiation of registered nurse
practice: Historical perspectives meet contemporary efforts. *Journal of
Nursing Education and Practice, 5*(4), 108–114. doi:10.5430/jnep.v5n4p108

Matthias, A. D., & Kim-Godwin, Y. S. (2016). RN-BSN students' perceptions
of the differences in practice of the ADN- and BSN-prepared RN. *Nurse
Educator, 41*(40), 208–211. doi:10.1097/NNE.0000000000000244

Montag, M. L. (1951). *The education of nursing technicians.* New York, NY: G. P.
Putnam's Sons.

National League for Nursing. (2010). *Outcomes and competencies for graduates of
practical/vocational, diploma, associate degree, baccalaureate, master's, practice
doctorate, and research doctorate programs.* New York, NY: Author.

Nelson, M. A. (2002). Education for professional nursing practice: Looking backward into the future. *Online Journal of Issues in Nursing, 7*(2). Retrieved from
http://www.nursingworld.org/MainMenuCategories/ANAMarketplace/

ANAPeriodicals/OJIN/TableofContents/Volume72002/No2May2002/
EducationforProfessionalNursingPractice.html

Nightingale, F. (1872). Letter to Dr. Wylie. Archives of the Foundation of the New York State Nurses Association (MC 19, Bellevue Alumnae Association, Artifact Box 4). Bellevue Alumnae Center for Nursing History, Guilderland, NY.

Nutting, M. A., & Dock, L. (1935). *A history of nursing: The evolution of nursing systems from the earliest times to the foundation of the first English and American training schools for nurses Volume II*. New York, NY: G. P. Putnam's Sons.

Officers, Boards, and Departments of the City of Cincinnati. (1914). Annual Reports of Officers, Boards, and Departments of the City of Cincinnati for 1914. Archives and Rare Books Library, Blegen Library, University of Cincinnati Libraries, Cincinnati, OH.

Pitts-Willhelm, P., Nicolai, C. S., & Koerner, J. (1991). Differentiating nursing practice to improve service outcomes. *Nursing Management, 22*(12), 12–25. Retrieved from http://journals.lww.com/nursingmanagement/Citation/1991/12000/Differentiating_Nursing_Practice_to_Improve.8.aspx

Powell, L. M. (1937). The history of the development of nursing education at the University of Minnesota. *The Alumnae Quarterly University of Minnesota School of Nursing, 18*(1), 4–13.

Research and Experimentation in Junior Colleges–Nursing Education: A Proposal. (1951). Archives of the Department of Nursing Education, Gottesman Library, Teachers College, Columbia University, New York, NY.

Reverby, S. M. (1987). *Ordered to care: The dilemma of American nursing, 1850–1945*. New York, NY: Cambridge University Press.

Robert Wood Johnson Foundation (RWJF). (2013). The case for academic progression: Why nurses should advance their education and the strategies that make this feasible. *Charting Nursing's Future: Reports on Policies That Can Transform Patient Care, 21*, 1–8. Retrieved from http://www.rwjf.org/content/dam/farm/reports/issue_briefs/2013/rwjf407597

Rogers, M. E. (1961). *Educational revolution in nursing*. New York, NY: MacMillan.

Rosenberg, C. E. (1987). *The care of strangers: The rise of America's hospital system*. Baltimore, MD: Johns Hopkins University Press.

Rosnagle, L., & Darrington, M. I. (1950). *History of the college of nursing and health*. Unpublished document (Folder: Laura Rosnagle). Archives of the Wedbush Centre, College of Nursing, University of Cincinnati, Cincinnati, OH.

Russell, C. H. (1959). *Liberal education and nursing.* New York, NY: Institute of Higher Education.

Schuyler, L. L. (1912). Letter addressed to Mrs. Joseph Hobson dated May 19, 1912. Archives of the foundation of the New York State Nurses Association (MC 19, Series 1: People, Box 2: Non-Alumnae, Folder 34: Louisa Lee Schuyler). Bellevue Alumnae Center for Nursing History, Guilderland, NY.

Smith, T. G. (2009). A policy perspective on the entry into practice issue. *Online Journal of Issues in Nursing, 15*(1). doi:10.3912/OJIN.Vol15No01PPT01

State of New Jersey 215th Legislature. Senate, Bill No. S1258 (2012–2013).

State of New York 2013–2014 Regular Session, Senate, Bill No. S00628 (2013–2014).

Stewart, I. M. (1950). *The education of nurses: Historical foundations and modern trends.* New York, NY: MacMillan.

Trautman, D. E. (2015). Moving the needle: What the data tell us about academic progression. *American Nurse Today, 10*(9), 4–5. Retrieved from https://www.americannursetoday.com/moving-needle-data-tell-us-academic-progression

University of Cincinnati Board of Trustees. (1915). Supporting documents of February 2, 1915 meeting. Archives and Rare Books Library, Blegen Library, University of Cincinnati Libraries, Cincinnati, OH.

University of Cincinnati Board of Trustees. (1916). Minutes from June 29, 1916 meeting. Archives and Rare Books Library, Blegen Library, University of Cincinnati Libraries, Cincinnati, OH.

Vena, C., & Oldaker, S. (1994). Differentiated practice paradigm using a theoretical approach. *Nursing Administration Quarterly, 19*(1), 66–73. Retrieved from http://journals.lww.com/naqjournal/Abstract/1994/01910/Differentiated_practice__The_new_paradigm_using_a.8.aspx

Watts, M. D. (2010). Certification and clinical ladder as the impetus for professional development. *Critical Care Nursing Quarterly, 33*(1), 52–59. doi:10.1097/CNQ.0b013e3181c8e333

Chapter 8: "On Such Teachers Rests the Future of Nursing": Preparing Faculty for Associate Degree Programs at the Mid-20th Century

ANNEMARIE McALLISTER

On such teachers rests the future of nursing.
("Project for the Preparation of Teachers for
Associate Degree Nursing Programs," 1962, p. 6)

Nursing in the United States is a relatively young profession. The first organized nursing schools were not established until after the Civil War in 1873 when the Bellevue Hospital School of Nursing opened in New York City and the Connecticut Training School for Nurses opened in New Haven, Connecticut. Massachusetts was not far behind when the Boston Training School for Nurses opened at Massachusetts General Hospital. These schools were based on the Nightingale apprenticeship model where the student nurse was placed on a hospital ward and learned by example under the critical eye of a nursing supervisor who had the same education but more experience (Lewenson, 1993). Early 20th-century nursing educators argued to move nursing outside of hospitals and the apprenticeship model of education but progress was slow. It was not until after World War II that nurse leaders began to take advantage of the rapid expansion of the junior colleges (which we now call community colleges). The arduous process of moving the education of nurses from the apprenticeship model and into the nation's expanding community college system required innovative thinking and a new, 2-year model based on education and not training. That model was developed as a result of Mildred Montag's dissertation while at Teachers College (TC) of Columbia University and became the associate degree model for the education of nurses to take place in the nation's junior colleges.

The advent of the associate degree in nursing (ADN) model for the education of nurses in the early 1950s was a watershed event in the history of nursing education in the United States. It remains the most common pathway into a profession that has three different entryways: diploma, associate degree, and baccalaureate degree. No other profession has this issue. The success of the ADN model has remained a constant controversy within the profession, and the repeated calls (Brown, 1948; Goldmark, 1923/1984) in the first half of the 20th century for a larger and more highly educated nursing workforce remain unheeded. The American Nurses Association (ANA) joined this rallying cry in 1965, soon after the astounding success of the ADN model became clear, by issuing the position statement calling for the baccalaureate degree to be the minimum level for entry into the practice of nursing (ANA, 1965). Reports on the status of nursing continue in the 21st century (Benner, Sutphen, Leonard, & Day, 2010; Institute of Medicine [IOM], 2010), and the entry-into-practice issue has moved to the forefront as the evidence mounts that patient outcomes are better in hospitals with a higher proportion of baccalaureate-prepared nurses (Aiken, Clarke, Cheung, Sloane, & Silber, 2003; Aiken, Clarke, Sloane, Sochalski, & Silber, 2002). But even as we see these data calling for better prepared nurses, we also see an insufficient number of nurses who can serve as faculty to accommodate the ever-growing demand for baccalaureate-prepared nurses. The lack of a sufficient number of faculty at all levels of nursing education creates a wait list for those who might enter the profession and move into graduate education (American Association of Colleges of Nursing [AACN], 2015). Without faculty, schools have no choice but to turn away potential nurses. The history of the education of nurses to teach in the newly developed associate degree programs highlights what has been done in the past to meet increasing demands for faculty. In this chapter, I argue that the little-discussed but highly organized efforts to prepare faculty to teach in the newly created ADN programs in the late 1950s serve as an exemplar for the continued efforts of the profession to provide a more educated nursing workforce.

The history of the development of this new and experimental 2-year curriculum that would take place in community colleges and lead to an associate degree informs contemporary efforts to require the baccalaureate degree as the minimum requirement for entry into the nursing profession. Once the success of the associate degree model became apparent, nurse leaders, particularly those at TC, moved quickly to begin the process of educating the faculty for this new model. Nurses needed to learn how to teach in this new model and needed to be prepared quickly to accommodate the rise in the number of community colleges.

This chapter provides a brief overview of how the ADN was developed and then explores the efforts of nurse leaders to educate the faculty for these new programs, which were opening at breakneck speed across the United States beginning in the late 1950s. These efforts included garnering funding from the W. K. Kellogg Foundation, which resulted in the Four-State Project (FSP) and the establishment of demonstration sites to provide clinical sites for this new faculty and resources for administrators interested in starting new programs. The development of Bronx Community College (BCC), not far from TC and one of the faculty demonstration projects in New York, is presented as the case study. The historical significance of the efforts of nurses to take control of their own education is illustrated by the proactive advocacy of the nurse leaders during the mid-century. By removing nursing from the traditional apprenticeship model and paternalistic supervision of hospital leadership, nursing education was transformed from a model of student as a worker to that of student as a learner and reminds us that nurses are in charge of their own education. These nurse leaders in the mid-20th century recognized that the ADN model required a cadre of faculty prepared to teach in these new programs and were practical and realistic in developing a curriculum and demonstration sites, such as the BCC. Their advocacy for educating nurses instead of training them reminds us of contemporary efforts to further the educational trajectory of the entire profession by seeking to require the baccalaureate degree as the minimal requirement for entry into the nursing profession.

BACKGROUND

The Right Time

The post–World War II years brought many changes to the United States as the country settled into a new and more optimistic period. Many assumed that the military nurse who returned from the war would return to work in the civilian hospitals, thus relieving the nursing shortage. But this did not happen as many of those returning nurses did not stay in the workforce but instead married and started families. This would become the baby boomer generation (Waters, 1995). Many advances in health care were the result of wartime experiences and nurses were called upon to meet the needs of society. The advent of antibiotics to treat disease and innovations in surgical techniques increased the need for qualified nurses (Orsolini-Hain & Waters, 2009). The combination of these two factors resulted in a healthier population and an increasing life span. People no longer died from ordinary infections. As people lived longer, the development of chronic diseases such as cancer and cardiovascular disease required more nurses to care for an increasingly aging population.

Along with health care, the American system of education was a concern and in 1946, the Truman Commission published its report, *Higher Education for American Democracy* (Zook, 1946). In the report, the committee suggested that at least one half of high school graduates in the United States should complete 2 years of college and the focus was on the community colleges, then called junior colleges. As a result of the report, community colleges started to receive support and attention. The ADN model for the education of nurses, as developed by Mildred Montag and others at TC, mirrored the community college's philosophy, which was to educate people in the community who would live in the community, and then, once graduated, would work in the community (McAllister, 2012).

With the assistance of the GI Bill, enrolling in college became a reality for many nurses returning from war service. More funding sources for higher education became available in the early 1960s with the Nurse Training Act. The post–World War II funding of nursing education was pivotal to the start of real movement of nursing education out of the hospitals and into the system of higher education in the United States (Lynaugh, 2002). In addition, President Truman signed the Hill-Burton Act of 1946, which included funding for hospital construction. This bill, also known as the Hospital Survey and Construction Act, provided federal funds for hospitals in both low-income and rural areas of the country (Dolan, Fitzpatrick, & Herrmann, 1983). Both the war and the depression had taken a severe toll on hospitals with 40% of the nation's counties having no hospitals at all. This was the first time an organized community needs assessment was conducted and the result was the planning of hospitals and health care centers in underserved areas (Lipscomb, 2002). It was also during this time frame that health insurance for individuals became more common. In 1946, only one third of the population had health insurance and the inclusion of this employment benefit resulted in large numbers of Americans with sudden access to medical and hospital care (Lynaugh, 2006). The combination of access to care and the expansion of hospital facilities increased the demand for a larger nursing workforce (McAllister, 2012).

The Right Place

It was during this time that the long-sought-after goal of moving nursing education out from the apprenticeship model of the diploma schools began to gain momentum. Montag's dissertation outlining the experimental curriculum for the associate degree model for the education of nurses was published (Figure 8.1). Through the influence of R. Louise McManus, then director of the Department of Nursing Education at TC and Montag's dissertation advisor, funding was obtained for the development and experimentation of the new, 2-year curriculum for nursing. TC was considered the premier place for nurses to learn how to teach and administrate. It was here that leaders from all over came to study nursing at the university level and, thus, for many, TC was considered the "motherhouse" (L. Fitzpatrick, personal communication, September 2, 2010).

It was Mary Rockefeller, then wife of Nelson Rockefeller who was the governor of New York and later the Vice President of the United States, who provided the funding for Montag's experiment. She was a philanthropist, an ardent supporter of nursing, and a close personal friend of R. Louise McManus. This experiment, called the Cooperative Research Project (CRP), took place in seven community colleges across the country. Montag was the director of the project and four of her assistants were well-regarded TC faculty. And it truly was an experiment. Montag proposed a new 2-year curriculum, chose community colleges as the environment, instituted the programs, and evaluated the results at the end of the 5-year project. Her evaluation methods included the ability of the students to pass the licensing exam and included a detailed survey of the administrators who hired these graduates regarding their performance. The report, published in 1959, showed that the students educated in these 2-year community college programs that led to the associate degree performed as well or better than traditionally trained nurses (Montag, 1959). This propelled the model into what has remained the most common entryway into the practice of

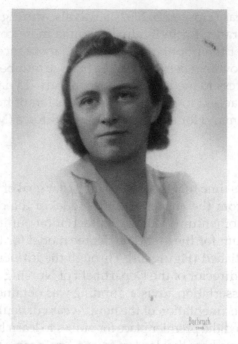

FIGURE 8.1 Mildred Montag.
Source: Mildred Montag Collection, University Archives & Special Collections, Adelphi University, Garden City, New York.

nursing in the United States (National League for Nursing [NLN], 2014a).

The success of Montag's CRP occurred over a 9-year period beginning with the completion of her dissertation in 1950 and ending with the published results of her experiment (Montag, 1950, 1959). It was so successful that by the end of the project there were more programs outside of the project than in it. The nurse leaders at the time, particularly those at TC, began immediate planning for the education of those who would teach in these new, ever-expanding programs. Again funding was sought and the W. K. Kellogg Foundation funded what became known as the Four-State Project (FSP), specifically to educate faculty for positions in these newly formed programs.

In this setting, just after World War II, TC's Division of Nursing Education dealt with the issues head on. Verle Waters was one of the first instructors in what became the first community college associate degree program at Orange County Community College in Middletown, New

York. She recalled that things moved fast in those days and that "some of the most creative thinking of the postwar period about the nurse's function and education came out of this institution" (Waters, 1995, p. 5).

This chapter now examines the way that nursing prepared educators to have the knowledge and skills required to educate nurses to meet the health needs of our society. The following case study uses the history of the associate degree programs, and specifically TC's newly developed program to educate faculty for these unique programs. In this way, the history of nursing education is expanded and readers are able to discuss the strategy and rationale for educating the educators. The initiative shown by Montag and others during this time frame reminds us that the education of nurses is the profession's responsibility and essential to the future of nursing.

Educating the Educator

An announcement on May 27, 1957, by the Division of Nursing Education, TC, Columbia University in New York City heralded a new program for preparation of nurses for faculty positions in nursing education in junior and community colleges ("Announcement," 1957). This new program was developed by faculty at TC in direct response to the success of the associate degree model, offered at the nation's expanding community college system, as a new and innovative way to educate nurses. The TC recruitment materials for this program outlined the opportunities for prospective educators and included courses specific to the philosophy and objectives of associate degree education. The first ADN program opened at Orange County Community College in New York State in September 1952 and by 1961 it was projected that there would be 62 associate degree programs in 22 states and an additional 8 to 12 new programs developed each year. The minimum personnel requirement for each program was one administrator and four faculty members. Existing programs were expanding as well. Thus, the opportunities for educators prepared to teach in these programs would be substantial (Project for the Preparation of Teachers for Associate Degree Nursing Programs, 1961; Figure 8.2).

During this time, less than 45% of nursing instructors had an academic degree of any kind (Lynaugh, 2006; West & Hawkins, 1950; Figure 8.3). Thus, the pool of available educators was not sufficiently qualified to teach in these newly developed 2-year programs. It was

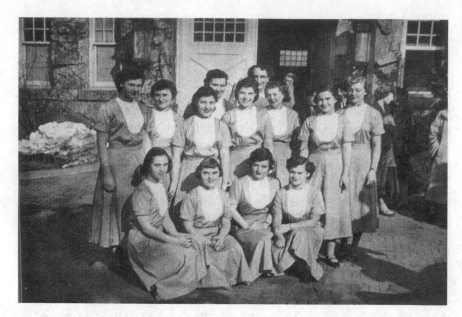

FIGURE 8.2 First nursing class at Orange County Community College, September, 1952.
Reprinted by permission of Orange Country Community College (SUNY Orange).

clear that the architects of these new programs needed a systematic way to prepare an increasing number of faculty to take up the mantle of associate degree education. This would help alleviate the nursing shortage and advance the long-held goal of moving the education of nurses into the system of higher education. TC faculty and staff were on the forefront of this effort. The process they developed and the resources they used are the result of the foresight and imagination of these nurse leaders and were predicated on the funding provided by the W. K. Kellogg Foundation and the ability to work cooperatively with the New York State Department of Education.

New York had a jump start in respect to the fast development of Kellogg's FSP by virtue of the involvement of faculty and staff at TC and the completion of Montag's CRP there in 1958. In addition, the Research Office of the New York State Department of Education put forth a report by a committee known as the Nurse Resources Study Group that identified the community colleges as the "most flexible of all institutions of higher education . . . and in a unique position to prepare much needed nursing personnel and in doing so also find new patterns of nursing education" (Hasse, 1990, p. 63).

State	Total number of nurse instructors	No degree	Bachelor's degree	Master's degree or higher
Total	10,477*	4,752	4,581	1,144
Alabama	99	66	30	3
Arizona	35	16	18	1
Arkansas	50	37	11	2
California	384	106	243	35
Colorado	145	35	93	17
Connecticut	286	103	115	68
Delaware	57	31	20	6
District of Columbia	75	10	45	20
Florida	98	59	37	2
Georgia	83	44	26	13
Idaho	44	25	19	—
Illinois	714	362	301	51
Indiana	243	119	112	12
Iowa	217	110	91	16
Kansas	182	102	75	5
Kentucky	90	51	34	5
Louisiana	115	55	52	8
Maine	82	55	24	3
Maryland	233	107	92	34
Massachusetts	626	321	235	70
Michigan	385	152	178	55
Minnesota	294	92	161	41
Mississippi	89	55	32	2
Missouri	297	118	138	41
Montana	56	20	32	4
Nebraska	127	50	62	15
Nevada	—	—		
New Hampshire	88	56	21	11
New Jersey	370	198	128	44
New Mexico	17	6	7	4
New York	1,238	496	533	209
North Carolina	225	170	53	2
North Dakota	68	36	29	3
Ohio	640	244	318	78
Oklahoma	74	35	32	7
Oregon	80	19	59	2
Pennsylvania	1,038	479	453	106
Rhode Island	46	15	27	4
South Carolina	92	68	19	5
South Dakota	83	39	42	2
Tennessee	135	58	57	20
Texas	259	118	108	33
Utah	52	15	29	8
Vermont	56	17	27	12
Virginia	186	105	71	10
Washington	200	73	104	23
West Virginia	128	80	41	7
Wisconsin	225	80	125	20
Wyoming	—	—	—	—
Hawaii	25	3	18	4
Puerto Rico	46	41	4	1

FIGURE 8.3 Nurse instructors and academics degrees held, by state, 1949.

*Reported schools only.

Source: West and Hawkins (1950, p. 78).

The compilation of events in New York and the continued involvement of TC faculty resulted in the implementation of several projects. First, TC would prepare students for faculty roles in associate degree nursing programs. The program opened in September 1959 with a total of 37 students: 28 for a master's degree and nine for post-master's and doctoral degrees. Of note, five of the students were already employed in associate degree programs: three at Orange County Community College and two at Fairleigh Dickinson University (Project for the Preparation of Teachers for Associate Degree Nursing Programs, 1960).

The TC faculty would also play a major consultative role for community college administrators who were interested in starting nursing programs, as had been done in the CRP that Montag had completed in 1958 (Montag, 1959). Staff at community colleges involved in the CRP found the meetings and conferences of value as they allowed for many to come together and discuss both the problems and the successes of individual programs and hence the means to include them was instituted when the grant from the W. K. Kellogg Foundation was developed. The work conferences held at TC were for all programs located to the east of the Mississippi River and were for those whose focus was on the teaching, administering, and consulting in associate degree programs in community colleges. The annual report from 1960 notes that the "main focus of the Work Conference was the enlarging of the understanding by the participants of the specialized areas of the curriculum and the teaching of nursing courses offered by a program in community colleges" (Project for the Preparation of Teachers for Associate Degree Nursing Programs, 1960, p. 94).

Faculty at TC held the work conferences annually for the duration of the FSP. These included general sessions about the community college objectives and philosophy, an initial discussion with the entire group, and then group sessions in specific instructional areas (fundamentals, nursing of mothers and children, and nursing in physical and mental illness). The committee for planning these work conferences included Mildred Montag, Eleanor Carlson, Barbara Hanford, Alice Riesman, and Sophia Yaczola—all part of faculty at TC in the program to prepare faculty for teaching in the associate degree programs (Project for the Preparation of Teachers for Associate Degree Nursing Programs, 1960).

One of the first ADN educators at Orange County Community College, Verle Waters, commented on the value of these conferences, saying:

> I mean we were constructing our own reality as we went along. Recreating the vision. Solving the practical questions that went with recreating this new vision of nursing

education. And since none of us, of course, had been prepared for these jobs, none of us had been in programs like that, there was a great deal of what I look on as being the success of those programs that derived from those get togethers [*sic*]. (Verle Waters Interview, 1989)

CASE STUDY: The Choice of Bronx Community College in New York

The need for a central demonstration site for educators in the associate degree programs became apparent as requests for information and assistance in setting up nursing programs came pouring into TC from community colleges across the country. In addition to providing a site for students from the newly established program at TC to prepare faculty to teach in the associate degree programs, the central office in Albany, New York, would serve as a clearinghouse for material pertaining to associate degree education. This was an age before the Internet so materials were centrally located and mailed out as requested. Additionally, a demonstration site would be a place to innovate, evaluate, and revise curriculum as needed and would also serve as a site for educators and staff from community colleges that were interested in starting their own programs.

The demonstration center was developed at the nearby BCC, the first to offer an ADN in New York City. The first ADN BCC class of 44 students was enrolled in 1960 and clinical training took place at local sites, which included Montefiore, Morrisania, and Jacobi Hospitals. Its status as a demonstration project put the college in the forefront of ADN throughout New York State (Communicator, 2010).

BCC began its teaching initiatives in 1957 and opened with 125 students on February 2, 1959, and thus was a brand new college. The college was located on 184th Street and Creston Avenue in the Bronx, one of the five New York City boroughs and home to several well-known schools and universities. The college opened at the former site of the Bronx High School of Science and expanded to multiple buildings until 1973 when it

(continued)

CASE STUDY: The Choice of Bronx Community College in New York
(continued)

was moved to the former New York University's University Heights 43-acre campus where it remains today with an enrollment of over 11,000 students each semester (BCC, 2012).

BCC was a natural choice for a demonstration site for several reasons. The recent completion of the CRP (Montag, 1959) and the rapid development of community college programs for the education of nurses added new urgency to the need for faculty trained to teach at this new and innovative level of nursing education. The compilation of events in New York during the 1950s, which helped usher in and contribute to the success of Montag's model, continued in the early 1960s with the assistance of the W. K. Kellogg Foundation, which had interest in assisting in the development of ADN programs. The W. K. Kellogg Foundation had a long history of concern about the nation's inadequate supply of nurses to provide care for the populace and how the success of the model generated the need for faculty. By 1965, the W. K. Kellogg Foundation embarked on a plan to "support associate degree education for nurses by focusing on the preparation of faculty specifically to teach in ADN programs . . . to prepare nurses for beginning teaching positions in junior colleges, and to provide consultation services to developing ADN programs" (Haase, 1990, p. 146).

The legacies of this project were numerous. First, the impact on the teachers in ADN programs clearly created an expansion of nursing education and ensured the quality of such programs. The ability to practice both teaching and administration in an actual community college setting was a major initiative and an important part of the preparation of teachers for these new programs. The curriculum required 32 to 40 credits and was designed to be completed in 1 year of full-time study. It included "courses for all students preparing for educational positions in institutions of higher education and in junior and community colleges in particular . . . and seminars and field courses dealing specifically with the problem of the teaching of nursing

(continued)

CASE STUDY: The Choice of Bronx Community College in New York
(continued)

and the development of nursing education curricula in junior and community colleges" (Announcement, 1957, p. 2). The program announcement touted TC's strategic position due to its long history of professional leadership in both education and nursing and its ability to marshal the resources of other departments and divisions in the school to support this new curriculum.

Second, the development of a resource center for educational materials was maintained at the project's office in Albany and was available to all faculty involved in these programs. The library was to be maintained after the termination of the project and it was noted that other parts of the country could benefit from this type of central repository. Third, the project participants noted the value of the demonstration centers such as BCC. These centers included additional faculty members who were free to pursue new ideas and experiment with curricula and teaching methods, a hallmark of the development of the ADN. There were opportunities for visitors interested in starting their own programs to practice with both faculty and administration (New York State Associate Degree Nursing Project, 1959–1964).

Additionally, the New York State Associate Degree Nursing Project published 16 research projects reflecting a variety of teaching modalities that new faculty needed. For example, cutting-edge technology in the classroom, such as closed circuit television, was explored in an effort to reduce the number of faculty needed to teach in the clinical arena. There was a concerted effort to conduct surveys of clinical facilities in areas where new programs were to be developed and to ensure the presence of nursing faculty on each campus months prior to the start of any new program. Additionally, the need to utilize the faculty effectively was always a concern, and multiple studies included the use of closed circuit television to allow more students per one instructor in the clinical area. Programmed

(continued)

CASE STUDY: The Choice of Bronx Community College in New York
(continued)

instruction was also assessed as a means to provide more self-teaching on the part of the students (New York State Associate Degree Nursing Project: A Final Report, 1964). Like simulation today, the programs offered alternative methods for teaching and learning and provided instruction in their use.

The advent of the ADN model for the education of nurses facilitated a new cohort of students previously unseen in the nursing profession that included men, older women, and people of color. The degree achieved the long-held goal of nurse leaders to move the education of nurses into the collegiate system of education, and it pragmatically addressed the nursing shortage of the time. As a result of the success of the ADN, faculty at TC, supported by funding from the W. K. Kellogg Foundation, moved forward with a new program to train the educators needed for programs that were developing at breakneck speed across the United States. This new program, started in 1957, offered courses specific to the philosophy and objectives of associate degree education.

Ultimately, BCC, the demonstration project in New York, enrolled more than 600 nursing students, saw almost 400 faculty visitors, and received visits from educators from around the world. Requests for visiting and for teaching privileges were so great that a second demonstration center was established in Suffern, New York, at Rockland Community College. The ideas created by the associate degree proponents had a lasting legacy on the role of the nurse as well as that of the educator. The development of a specific curriculum to prepare educators to teach in the new ADN programs and the development of demonstration centers such as BCC is representative of the ability of nurse leaders at the time to be both forward thinking and innovative in their efforts. The need for more nurses and the desire to move the education of nurses into the system of higher education at the mid-20th century required new ideas and intense collaboration with agencies such as the New York State Department of Education and the financial backing of the W. K. Kellogg Foundation as

CASE STUDY: The Choice of Bronx Community College in New York (continued)

illustrated in this case study. Contemporary efforts to increase the number of nurses in the workforce are still thwarted by a lack of qualified faculty today, almost 60 years later.

DISCUSSION AND CONCLUSION

The NLN, an organization for faculty and leaders in nursing education, singled out the faculty shortage in the United States as a key metric requiring focus as the nursing profession struggles with a shortage of sufficient seats for qualified nursing school applicants. Faculty, the backbone of the nursing pipeline, are essential to increase both the number of nurses and the ability to provide a more educated nursing workforce as we continue to respond to the recommendations outlined in the IOM report (2010) to reach the goal of 80% of the nursing workforce to be educated at the baccalaureate level by 2020 (NLN, 2014b).

So how do we, as a profession, educate those who teach nursing? How do we teach the teachers? Current requirements vary widely. In 2005, the NLN board of governors released their position statement stressing that nursing education must be research based and call for the development of new models of nursing education. They clearly state that, "We can no longer rely on tradition, past practices, and good intentions. Instead, recommendations . . . should emanate from evidence that substantiates the science of nursing education and provides the foundation for best educational practices" (NLN, 2005). This call, although presented as new, can be found throughout modern nursing history, starting with Nightingale's call for the trained nurse. The post–World War II milieu resulted in successful efforts of nurse leaders, notably those at TC, to move the education of nurses from the apprentice model of the diploma schools common at the time and into the collegiate system of education, specifically into the nation's community colleges. These efforts were based on the evidence that resulted from Montag's CRP (Montag, 1959) and led to the development of the associate degree model. The success of this model was unprecedented in nursing education, and it remains the most common pathway into the profession today. The consistent call for a more educated nursing work-force (Brown, 1948; Goldmark, 1923/1984) resounded with these edu-cators at the mid-century just as the similar subsequent reports do with educators today (Benner et al., 2010; IOM, 2010). The success of Montag's ADN model for the education of nurses precipitated a definitive pro-gram, again developed at TC, to prepare faculty to teach in these newly developed 2-year programs. The organized and focused efforts of these nurse leaders to meet the needs of nursing and society were systematic and based on the evidence from the CRP (Montag, 1959). It resulted in a formal program of study for the faculty that would teach in these new programs as well as consistent efforts to improve the associate degree curriculum. The ability of the innovative faculty at TC dur-ing this time period to work cooperatively with the New York State Department of Education and utilize funding from the W. K. Kellogg Foundation to develop the demonstration site at BCC was remarkable. It required collaboration and planning that was possible due to the concentrated and focused efforts of educators at TC and the ability to garner the funding necessary for the success of their efforts. It is rare in nursing to achieve large-scale change such as that which occurred with the advent of the ADN and the subsequent development of a curriculum to prepare faculty to teach this new model. Current efforts to increase the number of nursing faculty across all levels can be informed by the actions and cooperative efforts of these leaders at the mid-20th century.

ACTIVITIES FOR TEACHING AND LEARNING

1. Assess the reports on the status of nursing/nursing education (Benner et al., 2010; Brown, 1948; Goldmark, 1923/1984) and the IOM report (2010). Why are the repeated calls for a better educated nursing workforce presented as new?

2. Compare two primary source documents related to the three path-ways into the nursing profession. Contemporary efforts to require the baccalaureate degree seem to have been taken out of nursing hands as a result of Magnet status requirements and a growing body of literature demonstrating better outcomes for patients in hospitals with a higher percentage of baccalaureate-prepared nurse (Aiken et al., 2002, 2003). Financial issues in today's health care system seem to eclipse the larger issue of nursing's status as the least educated

of the professions as almost 60% of the nurses enter via the associate degree pathway. Even current efforts moving toward a "BSN in
10" do not address the role differentiation. Is there evidence that the
IOM's goal of 80% by 2020 does not address the remaining 20%?
Should separate licensing requirement be considered?

3. Consider who the stakeholders are in the continued efforts to require
a baccalaureate degree as the minimum requirement for the practice
of nursing. The students who aspire to become nurses, nursing leadership, hospital and health care administrators, and administrators
of diploma and associate degree programs all have motivation.
Consider what each group's motives are and what is at stake as we
move toward the baccalaureate degree as the minimal requirement
for entry into practice.

REFERENCES

Aiken, L., Clarke, S., Cheung, R., Sloane, D., & Silber, J. (2003). Education levels
of hospital nurses and surgical patient mortality. *Journal of the American
Medical Association, 290*(12), 1617–1623.

Aiken, L., Clarke, S., Sloane, D., Sochalski, J., & Silber, J. (2002). Hospital nurse
staffing and patient mortality, nurse burnout, and job dissatisfaction.
Journal of the American Medical Association, 288, 1987–1993.

American Association of Colleges of Nursing. (2015). *Nursing faculty shortage.*
Retrieved from http://www.aacn.nche.edu/media-relations/fact-sheets/
nursing-faculty-shortage

American Nurses Association. (1965). American Nurses Association's first position on education for nursing. *American Journal of Nursing, 65*(12), 106–111.

Announcement: Preparation for nursing faculty positions in junior college
programs. (1957). Gottesman Libraries Archive, Department of Nursing
Education, Teachers College, Columbia University, NY. Retrieved from
http://pocketknowledge.tc.columbia.edu/home.php/viewfile/73135

Benner, P., Sutphen, M., Leonard, V., & Day, L. (2010). *Educating nurses: A call for
radical transformation.* San Francisco, CA: Jossey-Bass.

Bronx Community College Website (BCC). (2012). History of the college.
Retrieved from http://www.bcc.cuny.edu/About-BCC/?p=College-History

Brown, E. L. (1948). *Nursing for the future: A report prepared for the National
Nursing Council.* New York, NY: Russell Sage Foundation.

Communicator. (2010). College celebrates 50th anniversary of Department of Nursing and Allied Health Services. *The Communicator, 1*(Fall). Retrieved from https://www.bcc.cuny.edu/Communicator/Archive/Communicator_SEPT10.pdf

Dolan, J. A., Fitzpatrick, M. L., & Herrmann, E. K. (1983). *Nursing in society: A historical perspective* (15th ed.). Philadelphia, PA: W. B. Saunders.

Goldmark, J. (1923/1984). *Nursing and nursing education in the United States: Report of the committee for the study of nursing education.* New York, NY: McMillan. (Reprinted by Garland Publishing, New York, NY).

Haase, P. (1990). *The origins and rise of associate degree nursing education.* Durham, NC: Duke University Press.

Institute of Medicine (IOM). (2010). *The future of nursing: Leading change, advancing health.* Washington, DC: National Academies Press.

Lewenson, S. B. (1993). *Taking charge: Nursing, suffrage, and feminism, 1873–1920.* New York, NY: Garland.

Lipscomb, C. E. (2002). Lister Hill and his influence. *Journal of the Medical Library Association, 90*(1), 109–110.

Lynaugh, J. E. (2002). Nursing's history: Looking backward and seeing forward. In E. D. Baer, P. D'Antonio, S. Rinker, & J. E. Lynaugh (Eds.), *Enduring issues in American nursing* (pp. 10–24). New York, NY: Springer Publishing.

Lynaugh, J. E. (2006). Mildred Tuttle: Private initiative and public response in nursing education after World War II. *Nursing History Review, 14,* 203–211.

McAllister, A. (2012). *R. Louise McManus and Mildred Montag create the associate degree model for the education of nurses: The right leaders, the right time, the right place: 1947–1959* (Unpublished doctoral dissertation). Teachers College, Columbia University, New York, NY.

Montag, M. L. (1950). *Education of nursing technicians: A report of a type B project* (Unpublished doctoral dissertation). Teachers College, Columbia University, New York.

Montag, M. (1959). *Community college education for nursing: An experiment in technical education for nursing.* New York, NY: McGraw-Hill.

National League for Nursing. (2005). NLN position statement: Transforming nursing education. Retrieved from http://www.nln.org/docs/default-source/about/archived-position-statements/transforming052005.pdf?sfvrsn=6

National League for Nursing. (2014a). NLN biennial survey of schools of nursing. Retrieved from http://www.nln.org/docs/default-source/newsroom/nursing-education-statistics/proportion-of-basic-rn-programs-2014-(pdf).pdf?sfvrsn=0

National League for Nursing. (2014b). NLN nurse faculty shortage fact sheet: Main obstacles to expanding educational capacity of pre-licensure RN programs. Retrieved from http://www.nln.org/docs/default-source/advocacy-public-policy/nurse-faculty-shortage-fact-sheet-pdf.pdf?sfvrsn=0

New York State associate degree nursing project. (1959–1964). Gottesman Libraries Archive, Department of Nursing Education, Teachers College, Columbia University, NY. Retrieved from http://pocketknowledge.tc.columbia.edu/home.php/viewfile/76006

New York State associate degree nursing project: A final report. (1964). Gottesman Libraries Archive, Department of Nursing Education, Teachers College, Columbia University, NY. Retrieved from http://pocketknowledge.tc.columbia.edu/home.php/viewfile/download/104788

Orsolini-Hain, L., & Waters, V. (2009). Education evolution: An historical perspective of associate degree nursing. *Journal of Nursing Education, 48*(5), 266–271.

Project for the preparation of teachers for associate degree nursing programs: First annual report. (1960). Gottesman Libraries Archive, Department of Nursing Education, Teachers College, Columbia University, NY. Retrieved from http://pocketknowledge.tc.columbia.edu/home.php/viewfile/73298

Project for the preparation of teachers for associate degree nursing programs: Second annual report. Recruitment Brochure. (1961). Gottesman Libraries Archive, Department of Nursing Education, Teachers College, Columbia University, NY. Retrieved from http://pocketknowledge.tc.columbia.edu/home.php/viewfile/download/102098

Project for the preparation of teachers for associate degree nursing programs: Third annual report. (1962). Gottesman Libraries Archive, Department of Nursing Education, Teachers College, Columbia University, NY. Retrieved from http://pocketknowledge.tc.columbia.edu/home.php/viewfile/download/106417

Verle Waters interview. (1989). Joan E. Lynaugh Papers (Box JL.0023). University of Pennsylvania School of Nursing, Barbara Bates Center for the Study of the History of Nursing, School of Nursing, University of Pennsylvania, Philadelphia, PA.

Waters, V. (1995). Second annual Mildred Montag excellence in leadership award: The founding directors of the first associate degree nursing programs. In P. Bayles & J. Parks-Doyle (Eds.), *The web of inclusion: Faculty helping faculty* (pp. 3–6). New York, NY: National League for Nursing Press.

West, M., & Hawkins, C. (1950). *Nursing schools at mid-century.* New York, NY: National Committee for the Improvement of Nursing Schools.

Zook, G. F. (1946). *Higher education for American democracy: A report of the President's Commission of Higher Education.* New York, NY: Harper.

Section IV: The 1960s and Beyond

Chapter 9: Professionalism and Practice: Neonatal Nursing and Newborn Critical Care

BRIANA RALSTON SMITH

> *The place occupied by the nurse in the care of the premature infant is of major importance . . . success in the field depends on special training. . . . It requires constant care in critical periods, with the ability to act as the occasion arises, and a realization of the fact that the care of premature infants often constitutes an emergency. . . . In the well organized premature infant nursery, the supervisor, the head nurses, and the staff nurses necessarily hold key positions.*
>
> (Lundeen & Kunstadter, 1958, pp. 37–39)

With the recent shifts in health care related to the Affordable Care Act, debates continue concerning how resources should be allocated to patient care, nursing's role in the delivery of that care, and the use of health care technology. The recent Institute of Medicine's (IOM) report *The Future of Nursing: Leading Change, Advancing Practice* emphasizes the need to analyze the ways nursing education and organization must continue to develop as well as the autonomy nurses should have when practicing to the optimal extent of their ability (IOM, 2011). Essentially, the debate leads us to question if and how we view nurses as independent professionals with qualifications to meet complex problems and needs in a broader health care system. The IOM report speaks as an example of the continuing debate that has permeated the 20th century regarding our considerations of nursing's dynamic role in meeting the challenges that the American health care system faces.

For much of the 20th century, the concept of the professionalization of nursing has been a point of debate as the definitions and requirements for what constitutes a profession, and subsequently a professional,
proved to be a moving target. Nurses have used a variety of means to
both attain and define their professional status. Early nursing reform-
ers and leaders sought to change education and develop particular
scopes of knowledge. They pushed for mandated licensure, and they
sought to develop associations and organizations that rallied around
their unique roles. Despite these strides, nursing has been relegated
by many to what sociologists Abbott and Meerabeau (2003) labeled a
"semiprofession" within debates about what necessitates professional
status.

As early as 1915, Abraham Flexner, the educator most well known
for his seminal study on medical education, addressed the National
Conference of Charities and Correction and proposed his criteria for
professional status of workers, addressing nursing in particular (Flexner,
1915/2001). In his address, he argued that professionalism be determined by specific criteria, including "intellectual operations with large
individual responsibility" (Flexner, 1915/2001, p. 156). He also specified
that professionals must "possess an educationally communicable
technique . . . [and are] increasingly altruistic in motivation" (Flexner,
1915/2001, p. 156). Although he hesitated to define nursing as a profession due to nurses' lack of individual responsibility, he did recognize the
debate surrounding nursing's professional status. More contemporary
definitions related to the professionalism debate include criteria that
share similarities with and build upon Flexner's. Although early considerations of the definition of professional adopted a broader approach,
such as Carr-Saunders and Wilson who defined professions as "organized bodies of experts who applied esoteric knowledge to particular
cases," later considerations of professional formation included more
particular requirements (Abbott, 1988, p. 4).

Abbott and Meerabeau (2003) cite sociologist William Goode's criteria for considerations of professionalism, which are based on requiring a body of knowledge, include specialized skills and competencies,
operate on a code of ethics, and focus on service to a client (Abbott &
Meerabeau, 2003; Goode, 1960). Regarding the status of profession or
not, sociologist Andrew Abbott nuanced considerations of professionalism by acknowledging that some veins of workers provide the framework for other professions to take control and ownership of a particular

field; he referred to this phenomenon as *subordination*. Abbott (1988) argues that nursing is a classic case of the lack of one group to attain full jurisdiction of its own practice as nursing creates an environment where medicine as a profession can control the complex system of labor. Current debates regarding the ability of nursing to practice to the fullest extent of its ability and the effect such practice could have on our American health care system abound.

Analysis of the ways nurses have cared for sick and prematurely born neonates throughout the 20th century is an excellent case study to inform how we think about contemporary issues in nursing and health care. In this chapter, the concept of nurses as professionals is explored using the case study of nurses who cared for sick and prematurely born infants during the 20th century. These nurses functioned in key ways that suggest that they practiced as professionals. Historical analysis of nurses and their care of critically ill newborns is significant because it reveals the ways nurses have functioned independently, garnering and growing a unique body of knowledge within health care, and have formed their own organization and associations to guide their practice. Using the development of neonatal critical care nursing as a case study (encompassing the care of prematurely born and medically fragile newborns), I argue that nurses' skill, ingenuity, and dedication to their patients influenced the development of neonatal intensive care units (NICUs) and ultimately reflected their growing identity as professionals with specific knowledge. The tenacity, skills, and creativity of nurses who cared for sick newborns in the early 20th century demonstrated qualities necessary for professionalization, often overlooked by those seeking to deprive nursing of its full professional status.

BACKGROUND

The development of critical care for newborns was an endeavor that spanned the 20th century and grew out of the convergence of the social value of newborns, emerging post-war technology, and the progression of particular medical treatment unique to neonatal physiology and needs. Nursing consistently influenced this emerging complex technological system we now understand as neonatal intensive care. Prior to the establishment of NICUs in the 1960s and 1970s in the United States, hospitals grouped sick newborns, predominantly newborns born prematurely, into units called premature infant units. Nurses who worked in NICUs built on the knowledge and skills of those nurses who worked in premature infant units during the first half of the 20th century. Overall, nurses who worked with sick newborns, whether in premature infant units or in NICUs, worked with a patient population for whom the mortality rates were too high and care increasingly included more complex treatments and machines.

Beginning in the early decades of the 20th century, the abysmally high neonatal mortality rates became a focus in public health circles. Through the efforts of public health activists and better sanitation methods, the neonatal mortality rates decreased (Meckel, 1990; Oppenheimer, 1996); however, deaths due to prematurity remained relatively consistent. Though the definition of prematurity varied, as some classified prematurity by the mother's reported gestational age, the national definition generally accepted by the Children's Bureau and the American Academy of Pediatrics (AAP) was any infant born weighing less than 2,500 g (Desmond, 1998, p. 159). Premature infants faced abysmal mortality rates, and a small group of physicians, nurses, and public health activists rallied to improve the mortality rates that plagued the newborn period. One component was the establishment of premature infant units where premature and sick newborns received care from trained nurses who had particular skills and knowledge related to newborn thermoregulation, feeding, and general care. Some cities established programs that transported infants to hospitals that had premature infant units (Lundeen & Kunstadter, 1958), which existed in hospitals largely from the 1920s to the early 1960s when NICUs emerged as places where sick newborns were grouped together to receive intensive care.

The premature infant unit nurses practiced with specific knowledge of newborns and their unique needs, and demonstrated skills the particular care of these babies required. The early premature infant unit nurses began to develop a distinct knowledge base unique from physicians and their ability to teach each other was necessary to the formation and expansion of premature infant units. These nurses' ability to teach each other and assess their patients became a cornerstone of their practice and added to their value in the early premature infant units.

Beginning in the 1960s, intensive care units (ICUs) emerged for sick newborns with both medical and surgical foci. Nurses used tenacity and creativity as they practiced and garnered the ability to assess their patients amid the new machines and changing types of units where they delivered such care. They knew when the machines, new treatment modalities, and broad technologies were not working for their patients, and that knowledge and expertise meant that they practiced with incredible autonomy during the development of NICUs as we know them today.

Historians have published relatively little regarding the care of sick and prematurely born infants in the United States during the 20th century. Many of the histories focus on the roles physicians played or particular disease processes. Perhaps, the most relevant literature to the nursing role in the development of neonatal intensive care has been written by nursing historian Elizabeth Ann Reedy who argued that nursing played key roles in the development of premature infant care between 1920 and 1940 (Ralston, 2015; Reedy, 2000, 2003a, 2003b). Although Reedy's work is seminal as we engage this vein of nursing history, physician historians comprise the majority of authors who have written about the development of neonatal medicine, intensive care, and the units where this care was delivered (Cone, 1985; Desmond, 1998; Jorgensen, 2010; Philip, 2005; Robertson, 2003a, 2003b, 2003c; Robertson & Baker, 2005; Silverman, 1980).

With the exception of Reedy's work, most of the published scholarly literature focused on the physician, and the expanding and changing machines and tools as contributing forces in the early units. Although both the physicians and the machines and tools did play a role in the development of care, nurses also played key roles. The absence of nursing in the current literature might reflect nursing's status as a "semiprofession" in the consideration of these authors, but a more complex analysis of nursing's absence might reflect Abbott's *subordination*. These nurses made the system work, but because they were so intensely foundational their story is often overlooked in the scholarly literature.

The story of the development of NICUs cannot be compartmentalized from that of the nurses who worked with newborns and garnered knowledge, independence, and trust, and formed their own organizations and licensure related to their particular practice. The history of neonatal nursing provides a rich case study to identify often-overlooked themes that should inform and shape our broader considerations of nursing's ability to meet patient needs and find solutions to problems we face today.

CASE STUDY: Neonatal Nursing and Newborn Critical Care

As nursing for critically ill newborns emerged, nurses practiced in particular ways that reflected the demands for professionalism asserted by Flexner (1915/2001), Goode (1960), and Abbott and Meerabeau (2003), including particular knowledge unique to the practice, responsibility for carrying out that practice, and organization and licensure for practice. Nurses who cared for critically ill newborns developed these aspects in their practice over the course of the 20th century as they built on and strengthened their practice and thus contributed to the formation of neonatal critical care in the United States.

Early Education, Particular Training, and Knowledge Development

Nurses who cared for premature infants laid the foundations for the formation of particular knowledge that they built upon and taught to each other. Premature infant units appeared in greater numbers in hospitals as early as the 1920s, and by mid-century became places where prematurely born newborns received highly specialized care.[1] One of the early seminal, premature infant units opened in Chicago at Sarah Morris Hospital for Children (Cone, 1985). As few textbooks existed relating to the general care of sick newborns, nursing students (or even physicians) received little formalized education and many graduate nurses learned on the job from more experienced nurses (Hess, Mohr, & Bartelme, 1934). In one of the earliest textbooks addressing the care of sick newborns, published by physician Julius Hess in 1922, such nurses who cared for sick and prematurely born infants needed to be "intensely interested"

---

1. We cannot specify the "first" premature station in the country, but do have documentation of one opened by obstetrician Joseph DeLee as early as 1899 (Cone, 1985). Though these stations appeared prior to the 1920s, more and more hospitals established them as shifts in American medicine health care policy changed particularly throughout the early decades of the 20th century.

(continued)

CASE STUDY: Neonatal Nursing and Newborn Critical Care *(continued)*

and willing to make "necessary sacrifices" in the care of their patients. They needed to practice "good judgment" and be prepared to meet "emergencies" immediately. Hess stated that the *"ideal nursing staff* for such a [premature infant] station [was], therefore, one consisting of a well-trained supervising nurse and a corps of assistants desiring this training, and who are willing to remain in this service for a long period of time" (1922, p. 146). His assertions reflect nursing practice that included responsibility and altruistic dedication. In the premature infant units, nurses worked together, learned from each other, and had a proscribed amount of knowledge to make decisions and judgment calls reflecting immense responsibility in nursing practice.

This acknowledgment of the particular nursing knowledge required to care for sick newborns eventually grew. In 1941, Hess and Lundeen published their seminal textbook for sick and premature infant care with a particular focus on nursing care. This textbook specified particular nursing knowledge and a unique role in care for the newborn, thus supporting nurses in these premature infant stations as important and responsible caregivers required to make particular judgments and have skills in certain procedures (Hess & Lundeen, 1941). The nurses who practiced in premature infant units developed incredible skill and were trusted by physicians and hospital staff on the units; they also took the initiative to travel beyond hospital walls to ensure patients had access to the best care they could receive. By the 1950s, a select cadre of nursing training programs existed and, in some programs, physicians and nurses trained together, side by side, to care for premature infants, thus augmenting each other's approaches to care (Wallace, Losty, & Wishik, 1950; Figure 9.1).

Responsibility for Transportation

Nurses not only had to work with sick patients, but also with new and changing technology in roles that carried greater

(continued)

CASE STUDY: Neonatal Nursing and Newborn Critical Care *(continued)*

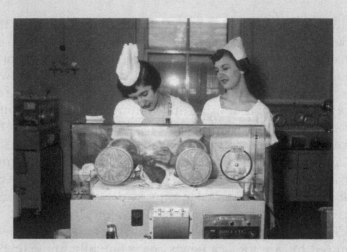

FIGURE 9.1 Staff and student nurses feeding an infant in an incubator, ca. 1950.

Source: Barbara Bates Center for the Study of the History of Nursing, University of Pennsylvania School of Nursing.

responsibility as systems to care for sick neonates evolved. In the same year the premature infant station opened at Sarah Morris Hospital for Children, Julius Hess published an article in the *Journal of the American Medical Association* outlining his new transportation incubator (Hess, 1923). This piece of equipment became incredibly important to the unit as transportation from homebirths and other hospitals was common. Units similar to the premature infant station in Sarah Morris existed in hospitals around the country, but not all hospitals could support the costs of equipment, staffing, and training needed for these units to run. Some nurses stepped into roles as transport nurses willing to travel between hospitals or to local homes in the area to pick up newborns who needed to be taken to a hospital unit where they could receive care (Losty, Orlofsky, & Wallace, 1950).

Some cities established formalized programs for newborn transport. For example, the city of New York worked diligently to establish a system to transport prematurely born infants

(continued)

CASE STUDY: Neonatal Nursing and Newborn Critical Care *(continued)*

from one hospital to another. Their valuing of the newborn and focus on saving the lives of prematurely born infants fueled their initiation of a city-wide transport system as part of a broader medical system consisting of public health measures, hospital units, and transport arrangements. The city allotted specific ambulances and staff to their premature infant initiative. Personnel consisted of nurses interested in the care of premature infants who received specific clinical training focused on premature infant care. They worked with ambulance drivers, also trained in the intricacies of transporting both the patients and the equipment needed, such as transport incubators and oxygen equipment (Losty et al., 1950). The nurses dictated care and were given the autonomy to make decisions based on their assessment expertise and knowledge of patients' physiological and medical needs. These nurses initially functioned without oversight and were trusted and considered sufficient to transport these critically ill premature infants sometimes for up to a few hours.

Nursing in the NICU and the Emergence of Professional Organizations

During the immediate post-war years as Hill Burton funds[2] flowed into the health care system, nurses found themselves caring for sicker patients. In the mid-1950s, ICUs emerged for adult populations as places where sick patients could be clustered together and cared for by specially trained nursing personnel (Fairman & Lynaugh, 1998). In conjunction with these

_____

2. Following World War II, the government invested funding, known as Hill–Burton funds, as a result of the 1946 Hospital Survey and Construction Act. These funds funneled into the system toward increasing hospital construction. Hill–Burton supporters argued that the program would increase access to hospital care for communities and families who could not otherwise afford hospital care (Starr, 1982).

(continued)

CASE STUDY: Neonatal Nursing and Newborn Critical Care *(continued)*

new adult ICUs, intensive care for sick newborns shifted from the premature infant units to new *ICUs*[3] where newborn ICU nurses worked with patients and played key roles due to their ability to perform excellent patient assessments. They built on the practices and standards of their predecessors in the premature infant units, but used those skills to care for a broader cadre of sick newborns. With incredible developments in pediatric surgery and increased surgical success rates for newborns with congenital malformations, nurses now found themselves caring for surgical and medically fragile newborns who previously had not survived. Their expertise with this niche patient population became a cornerstone of NICU care. Though some nursing schools allowed rotations in sick newborn ICUs, much learning was still done on the units as more experienced nurses trained new graduates.

Although intensive care became flooded with bigger and more complex machines, the nurse continued to play a key role in patient care and assessment. Not only did the nurses work with new treatments, such as dialysis and mechanical ventilation, they determined whether these new treatments worked for their patients and gave complex care as more machines were added and those same machines changed and developed. The nurses continued to be the frontline of care in the dynamic technological and systematic changes occurring not only in NICUs but also in the vast regionalization systems that emerged and grew in the 1960s and 1970s. By 1976, the value of NICU nurses in the vastly mechanical environments was reiterated in one important textbook, "Optimal outcomes are basically dependent on constant scrutiny of infants by personnel rather

---

3. Between 1955 and 1975, the specific title of these units varied. Some opened as NICUs, others chose terms such as *critical care units*, *infant intensive care units*, and *special care nurseries*. The term *NICU* is the common term today, but during this time unit titles varied for a variety of reasons and reflected social, medical, and hospital politics.

(continued)

CASE STUDY: Neonatal Nursing and Newborn Critical Care *(continued)*

than by gadgets. The crucial factors listed here are direct observations that can be made only by well-trained nurses" (Korones, 1976, p. 245).

The nurse practitioner (NP) movement gained momentum in the 1960s with NPs for adults and children emerging as ways to address primary care needs among the underserved and rural populations (Fairman, 2008). As shifts in medical education decreased the number of hours house staff spent training in any single subspecialty, the number of hours residents spent training in the NICUs also decreased. Such a decrease meant fewer personnel to perform procedures typically not assigned to nursing personnel including (but not limited to) examination and diagnosis (Sheldon & Dominiak, 1980). By the 1970s, the first neonatal nurse practitioner (NNP) roles appeared in response to the increasing need for providers in the growing NICUs of the 1970s and 1980s. The AAP required NNPs, as they were called, to have completed "a specified course in neonatal and perinatal nursing," and be proficient in particular technical procedures (AAP, 1977, p. 39). With the reduction in the amount of time resident physicians were allotted to spend in specialty areas during their training, NPs were one way such advanced care could be given. Many of the early training programs were certificate programs. Diploma and associate degree nurses enrolled alongside bachelor-prepared nurses to receive training in advanced nursing care (Samson, 2006). By 1983, NNPs received national certification from the Nurses Association of the American College of Obstetricians and Gynecologists (NAACOG), now known as the National Certification Corporation (NCC).

A group of dedicated NICU nurses worked together to establish the National Association of Neonatal Nurses (NANN) in 1984. After consultation with NAACOG and the American Association of Critical-Care Nursing, nursing leaders established NANN with the purpose of "address[ing] the educational and practice needs within the evolving specialty of neonatal

(continued)

CASE STUDY: Neonatal Nursing and Newborn Critical Care *(continued)*

nursing while giving all neonatal nurses national representation"
(Samson, 2006, p. 21). Such a nursing organization evidenced
the strong need for common knowledge and organizational
resources for nurses working with the neonatal population. As
nurses in this field had always required particular knowledge,
these nurses now banded together to form a national organization to strengthen their practice and solidify them as a subset
of professional nurses within broader nursing practice.

DISCUSSION AND CONCLUSION

The history of nursing gives us insight into the dynamic nature of nursing practice, how we might think about our roles in changing health
care systems, and fuels our imagination for how we might function in
more knowledgeable and critical health care teams. Nurses who cared
for premature infants laid the foundations for nursing practice and
knowledge that reflected the importance of nursing practice as a constantly changing and developing profession. These nurses developed
a knowledge base and taught each other the finer points of premature
and sick newborn care. Some nursing leaders, such as Evelyn Lundeen,
participated in the authorship of nursing textbooks as references and
repositories for the growing NICU nursing knowledge that developed.
With this knowledge came responsibility as nurses left the bedside
and moved out into the community to transport premature infants to
hospitals where they could receive care. They took initiative and responsibility for the infants en route without the oversight of physicians.
Eventually, NICU nurses formed a professional organization, the NANN,
to provide support and share knowledge. This organization brought
nurses from across the country together to share knowledge, give support, and advocate for the needs of sick newborns. All of these aspects
reflect the attributes Flexner, Goode, and Abbott and Meerabeau
claimed nurses would need to be professionals. These nurses practiced
with autonomy in particular circumstances, grew and shared a body of
knowledge particular to their practice, and formed an organizational
body that supports and organizes their practice to this day.

Nurses who cared for sick newborns across the 20th century were just one cadre of nurses who displayed those qualities. As evidence-based practice continues to effect change at the bedside in NICUs, nurses continue to both participate in that research and carry the knowledge base to assess and care for their patients. When we challenge ourselves to think about where we might adapt our care and health care delivery to the needs of individuals, communities, and populations for whom we care, our focus should not be limited to contemporary models and recent changes. The IOM's report *The Future of Nursing*, published in 2011, asserted nurses as key professionals who must play an important role in the imminent changes to come in the American health care system, and placed nursing as a key component to effecting change (IOM, 2011). Nursing's ability to adapt to broad themes and issues in patient health and the need to deliver particular care is not new. Nurses have traditionally met challenges directly when they identified patients who needed care within a system that might not necessarily provide them with easy access to needed resources. Such tenacity has always been inextricably linked to views on the nursing profession, its definition, and the scope to which nurses should be practicing in any given environment. Neonatal nurses developed a knowledge base and body of knowledge related to their particular practice and patient population, practiced with great responsibility as evidenced by their role in transport, and banded together to form national organizations. With these qualities, nurses who cared for sick newborns throughout the 20th century collectively demonstrated the qualities commonly attributed to professions; these nurses were indeed professionals.

Whether they met the definitions of "professional" at one point or another, we should never forget that within the roller coaster of professional practice they did their job consistently, they did it well, and they still continue to do so today. Although nursing has been in the center of heated debates, the label of professional did not hinder their ability to give good patient care. Such constancy in fact laid the foundations for professional practice whether it was defined as a grassroots movement or by broader consideration. Sociologists have published extensively debating the professional identities of nursing and what Abbot and Meerabeau (2003) called the *caring professions*. The concept of professionalism is considered by many to be deeply entrenched in gendered considerations of work. Others focus highly on the subordination of nursing to medicine. Although these arguments are important, I suggest we focus on the remarkable ways nursing did not allow its delineation as professional or semiprofessional (or even nonprofessional altogether) to hinder its work, growth, and ingenuity. Although the definition of professionalism has often varied and consistently excluded nursing as a whole, the nature of nursing practice has carried with it one constant: the focus on patient care and the ways nurses creatively and tenaciously met challenges to patient care. Nurses are professionals who not only practice in ways that uniquely identify them in the complex system of health care professionals, but also specifically have practiced (and might yet practice) in innovative ways because of their professional status. When we allow our historical lens to inform how we think about current issues in health care, we are able to question current assumptions and allow for more complex and nuanced evidence of the strength and tenacity of nursing practice and the nurses who have cared for patients throughout the history of American health care.

ACTIVITIES FOR TEACHING AND LEARNING

1. Premature infant nurses and later NICU nurses shared the ability to teach each other the skills needed to care for their sickest patients. Why do you think this is important? Does this still happen today in nursing practice?
2. In the case study, you read about New York City's early program to transport infants to larger, better equipped hospitals where they could receive care. Would this system have been possible without the nurses? Why was their involvement important?
3. Many (though not all) of the early physicians who cared for premature and sick infants were men. Why was the involvement and authority of nurse Evelyn Lundeen important when we consider the gendered impacts of the ways nurses were or were not considered professionals?
4. The story of nursing and the care of sick newborns in the 20th century is a snapshot of broader themes in health care. Do you see these same themes elsewhere in other veins of nursing practice?
5. Do you think nursing still functions with the kind of tenacity and ingenuity these nurses displayed as they taught each other how to care for newborns, transported sick newborns, and formed organizations? How so?

REFERENCES

Abbott, A. (1988). *The system of professions: An essay on the division of expert labor.* Chicago, IL: University of Chicago Press.

Abbott, P., & Meerabeau, L. (2003). *The sociology of caring professions.* London, England: Routledge.

American Academy of Pediatrics. (1977). *Standards and recommendations for hospital care of newborn infants* (6th ed.). Evanston, IL: Author.

Cone, T. (1985). *History of the care and feeding of the premature infant.* Boston, MA: Little, Brown.

Desmond, M. M. (1998). *Newborn medicine and society: European background and American practice (1750–1975).* Austin, TX: Eakin Press.

Fairman, J. (2008). *Making room in the clinic: Nurse practitioners and the evolution of modern health care.* New Brunswick, NJ: Rutgers University Press.

Fairman, J., & Lynaugh, J. (1998). *Critical care nursing: A history.* Philadelphia, PA: University of Pennsylvania Press.

Flexner, A. (1915/2001). Is social work a profession? *Research on Social Work Practice, 11*(2), 152–165.

Goode, W. J. (1960). Encroachment, charlatanism, and the emergent professions. *American Sociological Review, 25*(6), 902–914.

Hess, J. (1922). *Premature and congenitally diseased infants.* Philadelphia, PA: Lea & Febiger.

Hess, J. (1923). Heated bed for transportation of premature infants. *Journal of the American Medical Association, 80*(18), 1313.

Hess, J., & Lundeen, E. (1941). *The premature infant: Its medical and nursing care.* Philadelphia, PA: J. B. Lippincott.

Hess, J., Mohr, G., & Bartelme, P. (1934). *The physical and mental growth of prematurely born children.* Chicago, IL: University of Chicago Press.

Institute of Medicine. (2011). *The future of nursing: Leading change, advancing practice.* Washington, DC: National Academies Press. Retrieved from http://iom.nationalacademies.org/Reports/2010/The-Future-of-Nursing -Leading-Change-Advancing-Health/Report-Brief-Scope-of-Practice. aspx?page=1

Jorgensen, A. (2010). Born in the USA: The history of neonatology in the United States: A century of caring. *NICU Currents, 1*(1), 8–11.

Korones, S. (1976). *High-risk newborn infants: The basis for intensive nursing care.* St. Louis, MO: Mosby.

Losty, M., Orlofsky, I., & Wallace, I. (1950). A transport service for premature babies. *American Journal of Nursing, 50*(1), 10–12.

Lundeen, E., & Kunstadter, R. (1958). *Care of the premature infant.* Philadelphia, PA: J. B. Lippincott.

Meckel, R. (1990). *Save the babies: American public health reform and the prevention of infant mortality, 1850–1929.* Baltimore, MD: Johns Hopkins University Press.

Oppenheimer, G. (1996). Public health then and now: Prematurity as a public health problem: U.S. policy from the 1920s to the 1960s. *American Journal of Public Health, 86*(6), 870–878.

Philip, A. G. S. (2005). The evolution of neonatology. *Pediatric Research, 58*(4), 799–815. doi:10.1203/01.PDR.0000151693.46655.66

Ralston, B. L. (2015). *"We were the eyes and ears . . .": Nursing and the development of neonatal intensive care units in the United States, 1952–1982* (Doctoral dissertation). University of Pennsylvania, Philadelphia, PA.

Reedy, E. A. (2000). *Ripe too early* (Doctoral dissertation). University of Pennsylvania, Philadelphia, PA. Available from ProQuest Dissertations and Theses database. (UMI No. 9965552).

Reedy, E. A. (2003a). From weakling to fighter: Changing the image of premature infants. *Nursing History Review, 11,* 109–127.

Reedy, E. A. (2003b). Infant incubators turned "weaklings" into "fighters." *American Journal of Nursing, 103*(9), 64a.

Robertson, A. F. (2003a). Reflections on errors in neonatology III. The "experienced" years, 1970 to 2000. *Journal of Perinatology, 23*(3), 240–249. doi:10.1038/sj.jp.7210873

Robertson, A. F. (2003b). Reflections on errors in neonatology: I. The "hands-off" years, 1920 to 1950. *Journal of Perinatology, 23*(1), 48–55. doi:10.1038/sj.jp.7210842

Robertson, A. F. (2003c). Reflections on errors in neonatology: II. The "heroic" years, 1950 to 1970. *Journal of Perinatology, 23*(2), 154–161. doi:10.1038/sj.jp.7210843

Robertson, A. F., & Baker, J. P. (2005). Lessons from the past. *Seminars in Fetal and Neonatal Medicine, 10,* 23–30.

Samson, L. (2006). Perspectives on neonatal nursing: 1985–2005. *Journal of Perinatal and Neonatal Nursing, 20*(1), 19–26.

Sheldon, R., & Dominiak, P. S. (1980). *The expanding role of the nurse in neonatal intensive care*. New York, NY: Grune & Stratton.

Silverman, W. (1980). *Retrolental fibroplasia: A modern parable*. New York, NY: Grune & Stratton.

Starr, P. (1982). *The social transformation of American medicine*. New York, NY: Basic Books.

Wallace, H., Losty, M., & Wishik, S. (1950). Prematurity as a public health problem. *American Journal of Public Health, 40*, 41–47.

Chapter 10: Nurses Politically Engaged: Lillie Johnson and Sickle Cell Activism

KAREN FLYNN

I did not do this by myself. I have people who held up my arms. There were days when I was so frustrated and said I would give up. And then I do a bit of evaluation on myself. At times, I'm very hard with myself because when I went into this, I said, "nothing but the best is good enough for the patient with sickle cell."

(Lillie Johnson, retired nurse and sickle cell activist, in Armstrong, 2015)

According to the Canadian Nurses Association (CNA), "Advocacy involves engaging others, exercising voice and mobilizing evidence to influence policy and practice. It means speaking out against inequity and inequality" (CNA, 2016, n.p.). Advocacy demands action, such as "participating directly and indirectly in political processes" while acknowledging "the important roles of evidence, power and politics in advancing policy options" (CNA, 2016, n.p.). Seen in this light, activism is viewed as a form of "role extension, which is designed to fit within the scope of practice of a health care professional" (Duffy, Blair, Colthart, & Whyte, 2014, p. 32). This chapter explores the idea of activism as patient advocacy, using the example of Lillie Johnson and her work as an advocate for people with sickle cell disease (SCD). By making visible Johnson's sickle cell activism, the objective is to inspire and motivate nurses to consider activism as integral to their role development, and, by extension their occupational identity, as they strive to improve the health and well-being of the population they serve.

BACKGROUND

The scholarship on whether Canadian nurses are activists is generally framed in a dichotomous manner; that is, they are viewed as either apolitical or as "political novices" (Ross-Kerr & Wood, 2014, p. 291). Some nursing scholars take issue with the supposition that nurses are politically apathetic. As evidence, they evoke the history of nurses' mobilization on behalf of the occupation at the beginning of the 20th century when they lobbied for registration. By 1922, all the provinces had legislation, proof of the provincial campaign's successful professionalization efforts. Organizations such as the CNA and provincial associations, such as the Registered Nurses' Association of Ontario (RNAO, 2015) that lobby and represent nurses' interests, are cited as further confirmation of activism. One notable example involves the CNA, the voice of nurses at the federal level. The organization effectively lobbied for an amendment to the 1984 Canada Health Act after it was tabled in parliament, which allowed funding for "health care practitioners" (Ross-Kerr & Wood, 2014, p. 291). A remarkable achievement, the "legislation also made it possible for a provincial health plan to fund service of nurses or other health care providers on a direct reimbursement basis, as the services of physicians" (Ross-Kerr & Wood, 2014, p. 291). Other scholars emphasize nurses' labor activism, such as their historical and continued involvement in unionization and collective bargaining as additional proof of political agency (Kealey, 2008, 2014; McPherson, 1996; Richardson, 1998).

Nurses' activist practices extend beyond the profession to include patient care, and initiatives to benefit the general population. Canadian nurses have pressured the government to enact seat belt legislation, and lobbied for measures to improve safety in the home and the wearing of bicycle helmets. The involvement of a few nurses and their allies in the defeat of the Gimbel Foundation Act in Alberta during the mid-1990s serves as a cogent reminder that "nurses are often oriented to the public good" (Wilson, 2002, p. 30). The proposed bill "was designed to permit the establishment and maintenance of private health clinics, institutions, lodgings, and facilities for those in healthcare or education" (p. 31). In addition to the facilities being privately owned, patients who received care would pay privately for said care. Had the bill been approved, it would have drastically transformed the Canadian health care system, as "a single and public funded health care system" designed to ensure

Canadians "barrier-free access to medically necessary health care" (p. 31). Recognizing the implications of the Act on the well-being of Canadian citizens, nurses made presentations to the Private Bills Committee detailing its impact. The nurses' intervention, Wilson intimated, is confirmation they had "bought in" to the importance of political action (p. 32). Collectively, Canadian nurses continue to be instrumental in the struggle to maintain a public health care system that is based on need and accessibility, "and not on the ability to pay as a basic human right" (CNA, 2009). Canadian nursing activism is further fueled by the exigencies of an ever-changing and complex health care system in an increasingly globalized world.

The restructuring of the Canadian health care system and the concomitant neoliberal ideology has had, and continues to have, an adverse impact on nurses' ability to provide adequate and quality care. One manifestation of restructuring is the shortage of practitioners, and thus the implementation of efficiency measures. The reality, according to Rankin, is that "nurses are frequently working under-staffed and over census," which translates into not enough nurses and too many patients (Rankin, 2009, p. 279; Urban, 2013; Waters, 2015). Again, it is nurses and nursing associations that have been at the forefront of challenging these transformations. To address the "new public management," Rankin created "The Nurse Project: An Analysis for Nurses to Take Back Our Work" as a way to "dialogue about how to develop strategies for nurses to talk back to the authoritative ideological practices of health care reform," (Rankin, 2009, p. 275) leading to broad-based political action. Included in Rankin's discussion was the group Nurses United for Change. Concerned about the adverse impact of hospital reorganization on nursing practice, the group decided to take action. Following multiple scheduled meetings with administrators that produced no results, Nurses United for Change engaged in "more direct political action" (Rankin, 2009, p. 277). They went to the press and submitted a report to the local health authority (Rankin, 2009, p. 277), but their efforts proved futile. Unfortunately, a downside of political activism, or activism overall, is the potential for failed efforts. To avoid romanticizing activism, students must be exposed to all its dimensions, including the drawbacks, such as the lack of response by those in power to the concerns, or face repercussions. At the same time, there is a powerful message that can be gleaned from Nurses United for Change on the importance of and need for activism. When the health of patients and the nursing practice are being compromised, acquiescence is not the solution.

The defeat of the Gimbel Foundation Act and Nurses United for Change are examples of overt political action on behalf of the profession, patients, and citizens overall. To advocate on behalf of subaltern or marginalized groups requires a level of simultaneous self-reflexivity in terms of one's role development as well as one's occupation. In other words, given how nursing is constructed, a critical reexamination of its professional ethos and how it reflects, reinforces, and sustains dominant ideologies, and practices is necessary. For example, nursing educator MacDonnell (2009) argues that heteronormativity, which is entrenched in all social institutions, shapes lesbian, gay, bisexual, transgender (LGBT) interactions with health care practitioners. Simply put, because heterosexuality is viewed as normal, or as the default sexual/gender identity, nurses, whether consciously or unconsciously, pathologize LGBT patients. As such, the LGBT community experience various health inequities, such as "lack of access to relevant programs and services" (MacDonnell, 2009, p. 159) is intricately connected to how they are treated and viewed by health care providers. There are, however, nurses and educators such as MacDonnell who have begun to prioritize the health of and advocate on behalf of lesbians.

MacDonnell's (2009) qualitative study is insightful for what it reveals about the varied and multiple forms of activism, but also the need for a broader definition, and conception of "politics." A narrow definition of "politics" excludes nurses' political activities at the local or informal level which occurs though involvement in "community-based activities and nongovernmental organizations" (Vickers as quoted in MacDonnell, 2009, p. 159). Lesbian health advocacy was not confined to the clinical setting or the bedside, but in the classroom and the wider socio-environmental purview of health and policy making. MacDonnell's participants also worked with other vulnerable populations, such as "youth, Aboriginal, and immigrant communities," which often include LGBT people "to foster culturally relevant care, programs and services" (p. 162). The nurses, their knowledge about sexual diversity, and their involvement in other advocacy opportunities resulted in the development of "important relationships with interdisciplinary health and social service workers as well as police, politicians, and academics" (p. 162). Advocacy can occur in multiple sites—both on an individual and collective level—and students should be encouraged to think broadly about these various domains that do not necessarily fall within traditional realm of the political. That is, activism does not have to be linked to the legislative arena, state institutions, politicians, and political parties. Before focusing on Johnson's role as a sickle cell advocate in the case study, some attention to why students' role development must involve being engaged politically is warranted.

There is an overwhelming consensus among some practitioners, scholars, and professional organizations that, given the ongoing transformation of the contemporary health care system, nurses need to be politically engaged, which requires knowledge about "issues, laws and health policy" (Boswell, Cannon, & Miller, 2005, p. 5). The sentiments expressed by Boswell and her colleagues are hardly unique to the United States, but remain a concern for health care systems globally. The CNA insists that nurses make the connection between the care they provide and the "bigger picture." Thus, the holistic and comprehensive care nurses provide requires advocacy and political activism (CNA, 2000). Politics is a process of influencing those in positions to make decisions that would lead to the improvement of the lives of the individuals, families, communities, and populations (CNA, 2000). In addition to historical and contemporary examples of nurses' activism, information on how practitioners can prepare for political action was also discussed.

Although not the scope of this chapter, some references to nurses' ambivalence to engage politically on the level suggested by the CNA, the American Nurses Association (ANA), and individual scholars such as Boswell and her colleagues must be made. Heavy workloads, powerlessness, management inapproachability, anxiety associated with public speaking, concern related to retaliation, time, and an apolitical curriculum are some of the rationales for nurses' lack of political involvement (see Boswell et al., 2005, p. 5). The aforementioned concerns are legitimate and nursing organizations must address them as part of role development in tandem with empowering nursing students to recognize how their work environments are not only influenced by political decisions, but are also "governed by health policies that are political in nature" (Des Jardin, 2001, p. 614). As a case study, Johnson's activism, which spans almost four decades and involves both the formal and informal realms, illustrates the numerous ways nurses can engage in activism including the benefits and challenges.

CASE STUDY: Lillie Johnson and Sickle Cell Disease

In 2010, the Lawrence S. Bloomberg Faculty of Nursing at the University of Toronto awarded Lillie Johnson a distinguished alumnus award for her lifelong commitment to health care and sickle cell advocacy. Johnson attended the University of Toronto in 1964, where she earned a diploma in public health nursing. Upon receiving the award, Johnson, 89 years old at the time, evoked the nursing profession in the interview, as she acknowledged the insurmountable challenges she faced as a sickle cell advocate. Johnson explained that "when you have a dream, you keep focused" while adding that, "nursing is the best profession out there" (Fanfair, 2011, n.p.). Given how nurses are situated within the medical hierarchy, of which Johnson is acutely cognizant, her proclamation about nursing being the "best profession" is strategic and politically astute, and connected to almost four decades of being a sickle cell activist (Figure 10.1).

It was during the 1960s and 1970s while working as a public health nurse that Johnson came across patients with SCD, a life-threatening condition that is characterized by severe, unpredictable painful episodes and complications that can

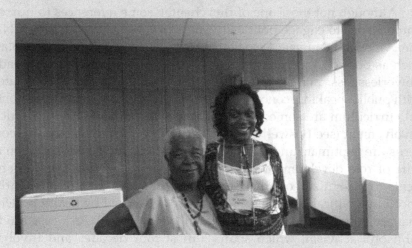

FIGURE 10.1 Lillie Johnson (left) and Karen Flynn.

(continued)

CASE STUDY: Lillie Johnson and Sickle Cell Disease *(continued)*

limit daily activities and cause disability. Regrettably, knowledge about SCD and its genetic and hereditary configuration was largely unknown—a reality, which Johnson recognized, with profound implications, including death. In an interview with Canadian Television (CTV), Johnson explained how during the 1970s, "The doctors did not know that these infants were being born with sickle cell . . . they were not testing if the gene was there . . . these children got very, very sick and we lost a lot of babies" (*CTV*, 2011). The next section explores Johnson's sickle cell advocacy efforts within the broader context of nursing activism and invites nurses working in, and beyond, the clinical setting to advocate on behalf of marginalized groups.

Johnson's activism is linked to her socialization in Jamaica as a child of deeply religious middle-class parents who abhorred individualism, and believed in and embodied the values of community. In Johnson's biography, *My Dream*, she wrote about her father, George Johnson: "He was always involved with the community and was a dedicated volunteer, preacher, choirmaster and social worker" (Johnson, 2014, p. 13). In a color-conscious, class-stratified, colonial Jamaica, Johnson's father, a teacher, advocated for school-aged children. According to Johnson, he ensured that "the English landlords did not keep children from school by employing them on the plantation. He convinced them to obey the law regarding child labour" (Johnson, 2014, p. 13). Her mother, Alnatal Johnson, also a teacher, volunteered at church and in the larger community. Etched in Johnson's psyche were the biblical admonitions to "love thy neighbor as thyself" (Matt. 22:39 KJV) and to be "[each] other's keeper" (Gen. 4:9 KJV). These maxims in practice meant extending love and care to others without concern for reciprocity, coupled with a commitment to community, create the road map that Johnson has relied on (Flynn, 2014).

Upon completion from the prestigious Wolmers Girls School in Kingston, Johnson's intention was to pursue nurse training; her father objected, telling her that "nurses have too

(continued)

CASE STUDY: Lillie Johnson and Sickle Cell Disease *(continued)*

much of a hard time" (Flynn, 2014). Johnson went to Shortwood Teachers College instead. She taught for 7 years, and while Johnson admitted, "I was very good at what I did" (Flynn, 2014, p. 152), she still yearned to be a nurse. At the age of 26, following her mother's death, Johnson applied to a hospital in Scotland, and in 1950, left her family and friends to fulfill her dream of becoming a nurse (Flynn, 2014). Johnson migrated to Canada in the 1960s and began a protracted and successful career as a nurse. Johnson noted that it was working as a community health care nurse with the Victorian Order of Nurses (VON) and the region of York, acting as a consultant with the Ontario Ministry of Health (northern region) and Maternal Child Health and Family Planning for Ontario, coupled with the leadership roles she held, that prepared her for sickle cell advocacy. Like the lesbian health advocates in MacDonnell's (2009) study, Johnson's activism was never limited to sickle cell patients, but included Canadian First Nation's people and immigrant women. It is important at this juncture to point out that belonging to a specific community is not a requisite to advocate for said community. Put another way, because Johnson is of Caribbean descent, while an advantage, demands more than cultural or racial affiliation. Knowledge about SCD, and the community it impacts, is critical if nurses are to advocate on behalf of this specific client population.

Knowledge and Activism

In discussions about nurses' activism, whether in terms of the legislature (formal) or the local and informal level, the term *knowledge* is ubiquitous. Whatever the domain, knowledge is paramount and is viewed as one of the key ways in which nurses can advance the interests of the profession while simultaneously improving the public's health (Hall-Long, 2009, p. 78). In preparing for political action, the CNA insists that nurses educate themselves, that is, they should "be able to speak or write

(continued)

CASE STUDY: Lillie Johnson and Sickle Cell Disease *(continued)*

knowledgeably" about the subject, which might require research (CNA, 2000). Nurses will also have to educate themselves regarding the key decision makers involved. They must also know at what level of government or institution is the legislation or policy being discussed. The realm of formal political engagement is not the only purview where knowledge is required. Johnson's initial knowledge about sickle cell was inadequate. She took a genetics course at the University of Toronto in 1980, which she pointed out was an "eye-opener and catalyst" for her "decades long quest to raise awareness of the disease" (Johnson, 2014, p. 143). Johnson then enlisted Graham Serjeant, a renowned SCD researcher, who was invited by the Canadian Sickle Cell Society to Ontario. According to Johnson, it was what they learned from Serjeant that enabled them to "start telling people about newborn screening for sickle cell" (Johnson, 2014, p. 148). In addition to organizing and speaking about SCD, Johnson attends conferences in the United States and the Caribbean about sickle cell to keep herself abreast of SCD research. Over the trajectory of her activism, Johnson has also collaborated with health care professionals, agencies, and a number of organizations to advance sickle cell advocacy.

A consistent and ongoing concern that Johnson expresses is the lack of or, in some cases, the absence of nurses' knowledge about SCD. Since nurses are often the first providers or carers who come in contact with patients it is imperative that they are familiar with the disease. To become effective advocates, there are a number of steps that student nurses and nurses can take to increase their knowledge of SCD. To understand the etiology of SCD, students might consider taking a genetics course. If, as in the case of Ontario, the nursing curriculum has yet to integrate sickle cell among the diseases studied, nurses will have to either take workshops, self-teach, or volunteer with the Sickle Cell Association of Ontario (SCAO). Nurses can further draw on the plethora of global research documenting SCD's impact on patients' ability to function daily (Anderson & Asnani, 2013;

(continued)

CASE STUDY: Lillie Johnson and Sickle Cell Disease *(continued)*

Caird, Camic, & Thomas, 2011; Cole, 2007). Knowledge of ongoing changes in health care systems, which also includes new patient demands, is critical especially in a province, such as Ontario that has a large and diverse immigrant population, many of whom are ignorant about sickle cell.

Patient advocacy is familiar terrain to nurses overall, and requires similar principles when dealing with, for example, sickle cell patients. Thus, upon acquiring the requisite information about sickle cell, nurses can begin to educate patients, families, and other health care providers. Nurses can also work with other institutions sickle cell patients have connections with, such as schools. Given the nature of sickle cell, and the population impacted, nurses must be thoughtful, flexible, and inventive. Fortunately, Johnson and the SCAO have the resources available that practitioners can draw on to aid in their advocacy efforts, especially in the education of patients and their families.

To educate patients with SCD, Johnson has developed an array of methodologies that are specific to her constituents' needs, gender, age, and culture. In addition to being sensitive to the physical pain associated with sickle cell, Johnson understands that it "carries a huge psychosocial burden, impairing physical, psychological, social and occupational well-being as well as levels of independence" (Thomas & Taylor, 2002, p. 345). Thus, she is sympathetic to the emotional and psychological distress that accompanies sickle cell, and works to avoid exacerbating what is already a difficult situation. For Johnson, dispelling the myths about sickle cell is crucial. Here, she describes a typical first meeting with a sickle cell patient, which can be adapted, or modified:

> I don't just tell people. I find out what people know, and I enlarge on it. I ask "Do you know how you get sickle cell?" Most people will say it's a Black disease. I will explain it to them. I have charts and use them to explain the genetics of the disease. For example, if

(continued)

CASE STUDY: Lillie Johnson and Sickle Cell Disease *(continued)*

> both parents are carriers, then there are 1 in 4 chances
> that the child may have sickle cell disease. Lots of peo-
> ple still believe that you catch sickle cell, or it's cancer,
> HIV, or sexually transmitted. (Flynn, 2014, p. 155)

The importance of helping patients and nurses understand
the biological aspects of SCD is intricately connected to the former's social location. For Johnson, that patients and providers
believe that SCD is inherently specific to Blacks has serious
consequences in terms of treatment and nurses' interactions
with the carriers. According to Johnson, "nurses see patients
more often than the doctor . . . if you [referring to a patient] have
an emergency and you are in crisis, and the first person you
see is the nurse. It's how she reacts to you; and how she talks to
you that will make a difference" (Lillie Johnson, personal communication, November 20, 2015). If nurses have internalized
racist stereotypes of Black people or SCD patients, their provision of care will be compromised. Johnson explains how patients
in crisis who seek assistance in emergency departments are
viewed as "drug addicts" because they require medication, such
as morphine, which "remains the drug of choice to achieve a
prompt analgesia in patients with SCD" (Niscola, Sorrentino,
Scaramucci, Fabritiis, & Cianciulli, 2009, p. 474). As with sickle
cell and other diseases, patients' experiences are mitigated by
social, cultural, economic, and political factors as well as by race,
gender, class, and other markers of difference. Research on
SCD patients can address some of these issues, but nurses have
to also be willing, as McGibbon, Mulaudzi, Didham, Barton, and
Sochan (2014) point out, to decolonize the profession and its
practices.

Cultural competency and sensitivity should also involve
teaching student practitioners, as part of role development, how
to be cognizant of their own and their patients' social location (race, gender, class, religion sexuality, ability, education,
and so forth). Attention to subjectivity formation, which is an

(continued)

CASE STUDY: Lillie Johnson and Sickle Cell Disease *(continued)*

understanding of the self and one's place in the world, and the role of social structures is helpful in advocacy. Nurses, for example, must see themselves as embodied subjects influenced by dominant ideologies that render Europeans as superior and non-Whites as "Other." Effective advocates recognize that subordination, which often occurs simultaneously, based on gender, race, sexuality, or nationality shapes social interactions, from which nurses are not exempt. Moreover, nurses must avoid the proclivity—especially given the absence of empirical evidence—to subscribe to a liberal discourse that assumes everyone is equal and has equal access to opportunities (McGibbon et al., 2014). In other words, when nurses adopt a discourse of "we are all humans," they are apt to ignore, as Browne, Smye, and Varcoe (2005) intimate, how "negative images framed as 'cultural' characteristics can become widely applied as markers of difference, particularly when health professionals have frequent contact with patients who embody manifestations of social problems and impoverishment" (Browne et al., 2005, p. 30). Notwithstanding Browne is referring to Aboriginal peoples, her example is applicable to sickle cell patients who are disadvantaged economically and are racialized in specific ways in the larger Canadian society that continuously denies the existence of racism, inequality, and White privilege. What does this lack of information mean for students' role development? Who is responsible for preparing them with the knowledge they need to advocate for, and, on behalf of subaltern populations?

Presently, according to MacDonnell (2009), there "is limited or inconsistent inclusion of critical and anti-oppression pedagogy in nursing education" (p. 165). For the aforementioned to occur, in conjunction with mandatory social justice, leadership, feminist, and activism courses, nursing students will need to be involved in transforming or revamping the curriculum. That students are involved in curriculum transformations is hardly novel; many women/gender ethnic/racial departments

(continued)

CASE STUDY: Lillie Johnson and Sickle Cell Disease (continued)

in North America were developed due to student demands, another form of activism. The benefits of understanding the integration of race, gender, sexuality, class, and other vectors of difference are not merely theoretical tools to understand, analyze, and explain the health experience of patients. How these markers of difference manifest materially inside and outside the clinical setting will be evident. Once students are equipped epistemologically, they will be enabled to critically think about how and why sickle cell patients are stigmatized as drug addicts, or dependent on some form of government assistance. Equally important, students will be able to analyze how certain ideologies and insights about sexual minorities, for example, are sustained and reflected in systemic structures, such as the education, legal, and health care systems. Upon graduating, nursing students should have knowledge of the historical, economic, and political factors that impact health care practice and provision over time. For nursing curricula to address the aforementioned issues, it will primarily be the responsibility of nursing students. The benefits, however, are enormous as nurses confidently advocate for marginalized patients, whether in the clinical setting or in other capacities.

The paucity of research on sickle cell patients in Canada is a major concern for Johnson. Until recently, the SCAO had to rely on research and publications from Jamaica, the United Kingdom, and the United States. Due to the absence of available data on carriers, requests to the Ministry of Health, Health Promotion Branch to produce relevant literature were denied. Johnson explains, how a "lack of Canadian statistics for the number of people who suffer from sickle cell disease has been used to deny us funding for programs, educational literature and other equipment" (Johnson, 2014, p. 154). Although literature from other geographical locations is undoubtedly valuable, scholarship that explores the uniqueness of the Canadian context as it relates to SCD is desperately needed. In addition to creating a more inclusive curriculum, activism can be

(continued)

CASE STUDY: Lillie Johnson and Sickle Cell Disease *(continued)*

epistemological in nature. Now that some data are available in Ontario, nurse scholars can engage in knowledge production with the goal to influence policy and legitimize sickle cell as a disease that is worthy of financial support. Similarly, evidence-based research on the epidemiological aspect of SCD, another mode of advocacy, can result in, for example, improvement in quality of life. The examples included here are intended to illustrate the varied modes of activism. While it might take nurses out of their comfort zone and feel thankless at times, a more formal form of political involvement is also an option. This type of activism is especially urgent due to frequent transformations in health care.

Johnson and Political Activism in Action

Even as Johnson provided counseling and support to sickle cell patients and their families, Johnson recognized from the onset that to engender the long-lasting outcomes that culminated into the law that led to newborn screening in 2005, support from a diverse group of individuals and institutions was required. The ability to collaborate and work with a wide range of stakeholders is essential depending on the issue and the outcome expected. To create awareness about SCD, Johnson and the SCAO spared no potential partnership. They liaised with "hospitals and other health agencies, churches, schools, universities, and colleges" (Johnson, 2014, p.152). To support their endeavor, Johnson and the SCAO forged relationships and partnerships with communities outside of the medical field that have supported them over the years. In the early years, teachers provided free space at the education center for SCAO's activities. Teachers also attended the organization's national conference, which met the SCAO's mandate of "informing and educating the community about sickle cell" (Johnson, 2014, p. 145). From its inception, enlisting the support of politicians was on Johnson's and the SCAO's agenda.

(continued)

CASE STUDY: Lillie Johnson and Sickle Cell Disease *(continued)*

It was Hon. Dennis Timbrell, then Provincial Minister of Health, who provided office space so Johnson could move the SCAO from her home in the mid-1980s.

Nurses have to be strategic in their choice of allies and partnerships. The daunting task of achieving universal newborn screening (UNS) was not lost on Johnson and the SCAO; they needed a politician to champion the cause, which they found in Mike Colle, Member of Provincial Parliament (MPP) for Eglington-Lawrence. As the MPP for the geographical that disproportionately includes the people most likely impacted by sickle cell, Colle was selected to introduce the private member's bill. He explains, "The Bill is a focal point for telling the story about sickle cell. And by telling this story we can have more people getting genetic testing and counseling, more resources and more comprehensive care for both children and adults" (Colle, 2012).

Indeed, over the duration of her involvement with sickle cell advocacy, besides Colle, Johnson and the SCAO drew on the support of "politicians in the different municipalities, and prominent community leaders such as Lincoln Alexander" who was Canada's first Black Member of Parliament. In lobbying for newborn screening, Johnson pointed out that "even the Black trade unions got behind it" (Johnson, 2014, p. 148). That the SCAO's first Board of Directors included Herbert (Herb) Carnegie was intentional. A trailblazer, Carnegie was not only a great hockey player, also but a successful and well-respected entrepreneur and philanthropist. To have Carnegie on the SCAO's board was added social capital. Other members at the time included physicians, social workers, businessmen, and hospital representatives. It is worth repeating that the success of any initiative depends on forming alliances with an extensive group of individuals, groups, and institutions.

Now more than ever, nurses, whether in a formal advocacy role or as practitioners, have to be attentive to the changing

(continued)

CASE STUDY: Lillie Johnson and Sickle Cell Disease *(continued)*

political landscape and the impact it has on the provision of health care. The dismantling of the Keynesian welfare state in Canada reflected in cuts to social spending and the reorganization of hospitals that led to the organization of Nurses United for Change is one example. Cuts to social programs also impact sickle cell patients who are often dependent on the state for some form of support. Johnson and the SCAO have had to be creative as strategies that might have worked two decades ago may no longer be applicable in the current political, economic, and social climates. The results are new approaches and an expansive vision, which involves partnerships with other organizations, such as the Black Health Alliance (BHA). Together both are committed to engendering awareness regarding sickle cell. Notwithstanding, the SCAO has formed alliances with the BHA; Johnson explains that "We don't want to just form partnerships with only Black groups" (Flynn, 2014, p. 162)—advice for nurse advocates who belong to a disenfranchised group. The propensity to only forge alliances with members of the group being affected is ineffective in the long run. As the example of Johnson and the SCAO demonstrates, much can be accomplished by forging partnerships with mainstream organizations and institutions. This is not to discount the relevance of groups generated by marginalized groups to address the specificity of their health needs. The SCAO's partnership with the BHA resulted in another of Johnson's recommendations coming to fruition: the development of a specialty center for sickle cell patients (Morgan, 2012).

Following an announcement in 2005 from then Minister of Health and Long-Term Care George Smitherman, that the government planned to increase satellite Community Health Centers across the province to improve primary health care and strengthen communities, the BHA saw this as a perfect opportunity to lobby for such a venue (Fanfair, 2012). The spring of 2012 saw the creation and opening of TAIBU Community Health Center (TAIBU CHC) in Malvern (Scarborough) to serve the

(continued)

CASE STUDY: Lillie Johnson and Sickle Cell Disease *(continued)*

disproportionately Black population in that city. Another of Johnson's visions materialized when the SCAO and TAIBU CHC, working in partnership with Scarborough Hospital, established an "effective and efficient" emergency department protocol for sickle cell patients (Fanfair, 2012). The inclusion of Scarborough Hospital in the broader sickle cell advocacy endeavors speaks to the importance of building effective and convincing alliances. Despite laudable and significant victories, Johnson insists that there is still more work to be done. For her, the inclusion of sickle cell in the college/university curriculum across Canada is the next step, which requires the support of deans, faculty members, and students. Again, it is Johnson's tenacious commitment to raising awareness about sickle cell that led Humber College to consider implementing sickle cell education in the curriculum.

Johnson has consistently and publicly reiterated her belief that nurses have a special role in sickle cell advocacy. She recognizes (based on own her experience) that nurses, as result of their profession, possess a number of skills useful in their advocacy efforts, which Des Jardin refers to as hidden talents. Nurses are "excellent negotiators, communicators, problem solving, and team players" (Des Jardin, 2001). Boswell further adds that, "Nurses regularly are required to manage challenging personalities, neutralize potentially unstable circumstances, and manage conflicts" (Boswell et al., 2005, p. 7). The skills are not necessarily innate, but can be cultivated, nurtured, and utilized as a component of student nurses' role development. Thus, nursing education must involve opportunities where students can develop their skills. The relationship between Johnson and Tiney Beckles serves as a testament to nurses' power and their ability to be influential advocates. That much of the SCAO's work depends on volunteers, Johnson has over the years developed a propensity for getting people involved in the organization. Beckles is an RN, and also a clinical instructor in the School of Health Sciences for the Practical Nurse/Personal Support

(continued)

CASE STUDY: Lillie Johnson and Sickle Cell Disease *(continued)*

Worker Program at Humber College North Campus. Beckles had a patient whose wife insisted that she assist Johnson in her advocacy efforts. Similar to Canadians generally, Beckles was also ignorant about sickle cell, and wanted to know more. Beckles decided to contact Johnson. Beckles joked that 2 months later, she became a member of the SCAO board, and, without hesitation, admitted that she "learned so much from Lillie" (Tiney Beckles, personal communication, November 23, 2015). Indeed, Beckles became one of hundreds of people that Johnson has mentored over the years, which is yet another example of advocacy. Once Beckles joined the SCAO board, she was inspired to become more involved in sickle cell efforts. She proved to be of tremendous value in terms of trying to incorporate sickle cell education as part of the college/university curriculum, which continues to be increasingly difficult as is explained shortly.

The scholarship on political advocacy is replete with examples of how nurses have been or can become politically active; studies on how mentoring translates into practice as exemplified by Johnson and Beckles could definitely encourage nurses. Johnson role-modeled for Beckles the ethos of advocating for a marginalized group, which led to proactive and concrete accomplishments. Beckles then sought to include others in the advocacy efforts at Humber College, which has continued without her participation. Like Johnson, Beckles, too, emphasized that critical care nurses can play a role in sickle cell advocacy. She insists, however, that nurses will first have to explore their own bias, which leads to stigmatization of patients before they can truly act as advocates, and begin to change the public perception. Beckles further underscored the relationship between education and sickle cell advocacy. She stated, nurses "need to be educated about sickle cell; if you don't have the education, you are unable to advocate. When you have the education, you are equipped to advocate on the patient's behalf— not as the person [who has] the disease, but as a person with a

(continued)

CASE STUDY: Lillie Johnson and Sickle Cell Disease *(continued)*

disease that can be managed, and help them to be comfortable" (Tiney Beckles, personal communication, November 23, 2015). This type of advocacy that Beckles and Johnson insist on is clearly attainable, but not all advocacy efforts are created equal.

DISCUSSION AND CONCLUSION

Advocacy, however, is not without its challenges. Even as Johnson has sought and benefited from the support of the state, its entities, and the medical profession, she is also critical of them. One cannot ignore the gendered implications of political advocacy in an occupation that is predominantly female, and where the fear of public speaking (Avolio, 2014) or an interest in public issues is cited as a reason for nurses' lack of political involvement. In a recent study on political activism and RNs in Ontario, the author maintained that "Nurses reported having a fear of conflict and public speaking" (Avolio, 2014, p. 93). While being sensitive to their fears, nurses must constantly remind themselves the reason for their advocacy efforts: the patients and the profession.

Johnson's ethos of community with its emphasis on working together communally remains at the core of her political advocacy. Thus, publically, she has critiqued the medical model, which remains physician centered as well as underscoring the limitations of Canada's medical system. Johnson's presentation to the Standing Committee on Social Policy (2008) exemplifies this. In addition to introducing a range of issues relating to sickle cell patients, such as language barriers, newcomer status, and suburban living, Johnson also provides solutions in the presentation, one that pointed to physicians epistemological limitations. In making the case for sickle cell specialty centers, Johnson explains:

> Outside of Toronto, when you go to Brampton, Mississauga, and the different areas, there are no specialists in the different hospitals who can attend to sickle cell patients, and we feel that this could be addressed at this level, that we do have

more trained people specifically. I know you can't do it for
every hospital, but I see that there is a problem when they
are turned away and not able to get [help]—especially those
who have just been discharged from Sick Children's Hospital.
At eighteen years, there is absolutely no care. Most of the
physicians are not too up to date with the care of young
adult sickle cell patients (Flynn, 2014, p. 159).

In this proceeding, Johnson relied on one of nurses' effective skills,
the ability to communicate a health care issue to politicians. Even as
Johnson recognizes the benefits of the Canadian health care system,
she boldly points out that the system was still lacking because SCD
was missing in the core curriculum for nurses or physicians (Morgan,
2014).

It is pointless to highlight the constraints of the Canadian health
care system in relation to SCD without offering concrete recommendations, which Johnson repeatedly does. There are several significant lessons that nurses can glean from Johnson's decades of activism. The first,
in no particular order or relevance, is that age should never be used as
a justification to remain uninvolved. Johnson was 88 years old at the
time she made the presentation to the legislature. She is currently 95
years old, and while her eyesight is rapidly failing, she remains involved
in the SCAO, with the objective to make UNS "truly universal, that is
across, Canada" (Johnson, 2014, p. 152). The second lesson, cultivating
a spirit of perseverance, is vital. Johnson's most significant accomplishment to date occurred when Ontario implemented UNS for 28 genetic
diseases, one of which was sickle cell in 2005. This accomplishment
was over two decades in coming to fruition, but Johnson and the SCAO
preserved, and remained committed to their cause. Johnson writes that
"Every year from 1981, we went to Queen's Park to get them to pass the
law until it was finally passed in 2005" (Johnson, 2014, p. 148).

As Johnson's example illuminates, depending on the issue, political advocacy and activism can be stressful and discouraging. Thus, the
third lesson is to focus on the minor victories; and the fourth is to continue to build a wide range of alliances, keep abreast of the changing
political and health landscape, and focus on the larger agenda. Johnson's
almost four decades of work educating a public about the symptoms
and implications of the hereditary disorder have not gone unnoticed.
In addition to the distinguished alumnus award from the Lawrence S.

Bloomberg Faculty of Nursing at the University of Toronto, Johnson has been the recipient of numerous awards and certificates of recognition. Perhaps, the most prestigious has been the Order of Ontario (2011)—the province's loftiest official honor which was created in 1986 and recognizes the highest level of individual excellence and achievement in any field. The fifth lesson is that, despite insurmountable challenges, there are moments when advocacy can be rewarding. The final lesson relates to age; people often express surprise that Johnson, given her age, has remained active. When asked about her age, she advises: "Don't let your age slow you down; if your body and mind tell you that you can do it, you'll do it" (Flynn, 2014, p. 164).

ACTIVITIES FOR TEACHING AND LEARNING

1. Identify a current issue that is impacting nurses, and write your state representative about it.
2. Identify an issue in nursing that you are passionate about, and use social media to raise awareness about it.
3. Create a petition to get support for a social justice course.

REFERENCES

Anderson, M., & Asnani, M. (2013). "You Just Have to Live With It": Coping with sickle cell disease in Jamaica. *Qualitative Health Research, 23*(5), 655–664.

Armstrong, N. (2015). Community stalwart, Lillie Johnson, launches her memoir. *Pride Magazine.* Retrieved from http://pridenews.ca

Avolio, C. D. (2014). Political advocacy: Beliefs and practices of registered nurses. *Electronic Theses and Dissertations.* Retrieved from http://scholar.uwindsor.ca/cgi/viewcontent.cgi?article=6063&context=etd

Boswell, C., Cannon, S., & Miller, J. (2005). Nurses' political involvement: Responsibility versus privilege. *Journal of Professional Nursing, 21*(1), 5–8.

Browne, A., Smye, V., & Varcoe, C. (2005). The relevance of post-colonial theoretical perspectives to research in Aboriginal health. *Canadian Journal of Nursing Research, 37*(4), 16–37.

Caird, H., Camic, P., & Thomas, V. (2011). The lives of adults over 30 living with sickle cell disorder. *British Journal of Health Psychology, 16*(3), 542–558.

Canadian Nurses Association. (2000). Nursing is a political act: The bigger picture. Retrieved from https://www.cna-aiic.ca/~/media/cna/page -content/pdf-en/nursing_political_act_may_2000_e.pdf?la=en

Canadian Nurses Association. (2009). Position statement: Nursing leadership. Retrieved from https://www.cna-aiic.ca/~/media/cna/page-content/pdf -en/nursing-leadership_position-statement.pdf?la=en

Canadian Nurses Association. (2016). Advocacy. Retrieved from https://www .cna-aiic.ca/en/advocacy

Cole, P. (2007). Black women and sickle cell disease: Implications for mental health disparities research. *Californian Journal of Health Promotion, 5,* 24–39.

Colle, M. (2012). MPP re-introduces Bill 105 to improve sickle cell care in Ontario. Retrieved from http://sicklecellanemia.ca/pdf/bill_105_press_ release.pdf

Canadian Television (CTV). (2011, January 30). Sickle cell disease activist honoured by Ontario. Retrieved from http://toronto.ctvnews.ca/sickle-cell -disease-activist-honoured-by-ontario-1.601811#ixzz2LsoJqE1X%29

Des Jardin, K. (2001). Political involvement in nursing: Politics, ethics and strategic action. *AORN Journal, 74*(5), 613–622.

Duffy, K., Blair, V., Colthart, I., & Whyte, L. (2014). Role development: Barriers, enablers and the function of a national organization. *Nursing Management, 21*(3), 31–37.

Fanfair, R. (2011, December, 12). Lillie Johnson honoured for work in nursing. *Share Newspaper.* Retrieved from http://sharenews.com

Fanfair, R. (2012, June 27). Malvern Health Centre providing prompt care for sickle cell sufferers. *Share Newspaper.* Retrieved from http://sharenews.com/ malvern-health-centre-providing-prompt-care-for-sickle-cell-sufferers

Flynn, K. (2014). "You need to press on": Lillie Johnson as a pragmatic public intellectual. *Palimpsest: A Journal on Women, Gender, and the Black International, 3*(2), 148–169.

Hall-Long, B. (2009). Nursing and public policy: A tool for excellence in education, practice and research. *Nurses Outlook, 57,* 78–83.

Johnson, L. (2014). *My dream.* Toronto, ON, Canada: Toronto Hakka Seniors Association.

Kealey, L. (1998). No more "yes girls": Labour activism among New Brunswick nurses, 1964 to 1981. *Acadiensis, 37*(2), 3–17.

Kealey, L. (2014). A life in history: Activism and scholarship. *Canadian Historical Review, 95*(1), 78–96.

MacDonnell, J. A. (2009). Fostering nurses' political knowledges and practices: Education and political activation in relation to lesbian health. *Advances in Nursing Science, 32*(2), 158–172.

McGibbon, E., Mulaudzi, F. M., Didham, P., Barton, S., & Sochan, A. (2014). Toward decolonizing nursing: The colonization of nursing and strategies for increasing the counter-narrative. *Nursing Inquiry, 3*, 179–191.

McPherson, K. M. (1996). *Bedside matters: The transformation of Canadian Nursing, 1900–1990*. Toronto, ON, Canada: University of Toronto Press.

Morgan, C. J. (2012, June 13). Institutions need to develop protocol for sickle cell disease. *Share Newspaper*. Retrieved from http://sharenews.com

Morgan, C. J. (2014, September 24). Lillie Johnson has been a sickle cell champion. *Share Newspaper*. Retrieved from http://sharenews.com

Niscola, P., Sorrentino, F., Scaramucci, L., Fabritiis, P., & Cianciulli, P. (2009). Pain syndromes in sickle cell disease: An update. *American Academy of Pain Medicine, 10*(3), 470–480.

Rankin, J. M. (2009). The nurse project: An analysis for nurses to take back our work. *Nursing Inquiry, 16*(4), 275–286.

Registered Nurses' Association of Ontario. (2015). Taking Action: A toolkit for becoming politically involved. Retrieved from http://rnao.ca/policy/polit ical-action/political-action-information-kit

Richardson, S. (1998). Political women, professional nurses, and the creation of Alberta's District Nursing Service, 1919–1925. *Nursing History Review, 6*, 25–50.

Ross-Kerr, J. C., & Wood, M. J. (2014). *Canadian nursing: Issues and perspectives* (5th ed.). Toronto, ON, Canada: Elsevier Canada.

Standing Committee on Social Policy. (2008, October 27). Bill 97: Increasing Access to Qualified Health Professionals for Ontarians Act, 2008. Retrieved from http://www.ontla.on.ca/committee-proceedings/transcripts/files_ html/27-OCT-2008_SP014.htm

Thomas, V. J., & Taylor, L. M. (2002). The psychosocial experience of people with sickle cell disease and its impact on quality of life. *British Journal of Health Psychology, 7*(3), 345–363.

Urban, A. (2013). Coercion over time: RN taking on the hospitals problem as their problem. *Journal of Nursing Heterodoxy, 1*(1), 4–7. Retrieved from http://www.journalofnursingheterodoxy.com/?p=193

Waters, N. (2015). Towards an institutional counter-cartography of nurses' wound work. *Journal of Sociology & Social Welfare*, 42(2), 127–156.

Wilson, D. M. (2002). Testing a theory of political development by comparing the political action of nurses and nonnurses. *Nursing Outlook*, 50(1), 30–34.

Chapter 11: Health Care as Women's Rights: The Maternity Care Coalition—The Philadelphia Story

LINDA TINA MALDONADO
AND BARBRA MANN WALL

We are doing things differently, but effectively. There's not just one way to get change (L. Maldonado, personal communication, December 1, 2012).

(Dorothy Jordan, Maternity Care Coalition's Lead
Community Advocate in the 1970–1980s)

The notion of active community involvement in the process of obtaining and achieving health care equity is an area getting much attention both in academia and health-related research. Nurses have historically been advocates for various communities and their health needs. As history shows, however, these communities did not always have a voice in the process of access to health services. Often, a community of lower socio-economic status lived relatively dependent on and invisible to the charity of those in economic and political power. Nursing has long been a voice for these communities and has performed this type of advocacy work by negotiating with those in power. This chapter demonstrates how nurses have been consistently involved in the ever-changing and politically charged domain of women's health. One central theme in women's health is reproductive health and reproductive control. This chapter explores the establishment of the Maternity Care Coalition (MCC) in West Philadelphia in the 1980s, focusing on the work of its early advocates and its role in the local community. As this study reveals, women's reproductive health is highly dependent upon the sociopolitical contexts where it is operationalized, and this has significant implications for nurses trying to provide the best care within the charged political arena of women's health today.

BACKGROUND

An Early Struggle

After the death of Sadie Sachs, a patient she had tended several times, Margaret Sanger (1938) wrote, "I was finished with palliatives and superficial cures" (p. 92). At that time, she "renounced nursing forever" (p. 107). Sanger wrote these words in her *An Autobiography* in 1938 to express her dismay over her inability to make a difference in many women's lives. She witnessed countless numbers of women who were dying after having faced a multitude of problems with too many childbirths and too many children to care for. Sanger's writings often highlighted real women and their children whom she saw dying daily, and she wanted to do something about it. She became the most famous nurse to advocate for contraception, although, by the time of her writing, she had rejected nursing in favor of a broader socialist agenda. Still, in Lynaugh's (1991) words, it was Sanger who "made birth control a worldwide, feminist issue. . . . And for her, the answer was knowledge and health care for all the people, not just the fortunate few" (p. 125).

Nurses have historically cared not only for the "fortunate few" but also for people from all social classes. Yet this vision of "health care for all," especially in regard to women's reproductive services, is under threat today. The Patient Protection and Affordable Care Act of 2010 has been a major factor in improving the health of women. The U.S. Supreme Court's landmark case *Burwell v. Hobby Lobby Stores* (2014), however, ruled that private company employers, because of their religious beliefs, could opt out of paying for health insurance for contraceptive coverage to their workers. An issue of major debate is whether or not they have the constitutional right to impose that belief on hundreds of women employees who do not have the same beliefs.

In the 1870s, newspapers blatantly advertised contraceptives as pharmaceutical products. This changed in 1873 when the federal Comstock Law for bade the trade and circulation of literature considered "obscene" and articles that were "immoral" (About.com, 2016).

Those who distributed pornography and also birth control literature were prosecuted. By the early 20th century, however, Sanger had begun her lifelong crusade to bring birth control to women. At the same time, government leaders such as Theodore Roosevelt were observing the decline of fertility in the United States, and they reacted with alarm over what they called "race suicide." In this view, White Anglo Saxon Protestants were dying out, and religious and political leaders presented contraception and abortion as not only illegal but also unsafe. Nursing leaders at that time typically were uninterested in details of women's reproductive lives. Historian Sandra Lewenson (1993) has described their support instead for woman's suffrage, which would empower them toward professionalization. Professionalization, not women's reproductive rights, was their main agenda.

The Judicial System Weighs In

The year 1936 witnessed a major change when a lower court decision removed federal bans on birth control distribution. It did so by amending the Comstock Act's label of birth control literature as no longer obscene. Physicians began to prescribe contraceptives to their patients, but because the devices did not require physicians to fit the woman, visiting nurses helped in this process (Schoen, 2005).

After World War II, the topic of birth control became a more acceptable topic for debate, but it was not until 1965, in *Griswold v. Connecticut* (1965), that the Supreme Court ruled contraception legal based on the Constitutional right to privacy. The same rationale was used in 1973 in *Roe v. Wade* (1973). The thinking was that choosing to have an abortion was a private decision between the woman and her doctor. To Justice Harry Blackmun, who wrote the majority opinion, and to the many physicians who supported the ruling, aborting a fetus was a medical decision. Thus, *Roe v. Wade* was not a women's rights issue but instead supported physicians' arguments.

The Long Civil Rights Road to Reproductive Health Equity

In the 1970s, women's rights became a larger issue for policy development and professional practice, and at this time nurses became more active. The women's health movement came into its own under the wings of the feminist movement and the pivotal era of the 1960s protests. The 1960s, with iconic images and wide ranging representations of protest and dissatisfaction toward almost every public and private facet of American society, were a critical tine for understanding the power, complexities, and tensions of the women's health movement. In particular, the decade set a foundational stage for the highly visible, powerful, and enduring intersections of race, class, and gender.

As women called for equality, democracy, and the right to claim ownership of their bodies, their health and its management became an important focal point. Despite its outward appearance of purpose, that of benefiting women, the women's health movement was fractured along its way both in purpose and composition. In spite of successfully building on the momentum of the Civil Rights movement, White feminists had to confront a series of strong backlashes from minority- and working-class women who clearly voiced their perceived lack of representation within the larger movement. Women of various colors and classes expressed very different kinds of concerns than their White, middle-to-upper-class sisters. Thus, this chapter also describes other women's voices and concerns that birthed a movement within a movement as Black, Latina, and other representatives of women came forward with their stories of societal discrimination and displacement. This was a period that witnessed Black feminists, middle-class White women, and radical youth intersecting with each other as well as a newly developing political Right (Hewitt, 2010).

Before the women's health movement took center stage, feminists were primarily concerned with achieving a sense of equality with the opposite sex across political, social, and labor issues. Black feminists, on the other hand, focused on articulating their race, gender, and class identities as interconnected. Emerging from the Civil Rights movement cycle of protest, but also at the same time as the predominantly White women's movement, Black feminists attempted to simultaneously define a collective identity and establish organizations that encompassed their rights as both Blacks and women (Springer, 2005). This emergence of Black feminism with its myriad of collective voices served as an important seed for Black women and other women of color in the larger women's health movement.

The 1960s' turbulence also witnessed a new generation of Americans expressing their dismay that the wealthiest, most powerful nation in the world could not adequately provide for its own citizens and sought other solutions. Michael Harrington's *The Other America* reminded a generation reared in relative prosperity of the hidden poverty that still crippled the lives of many Americans (Harrington, 1962). Young Black southern Civil Rights workers founded the Student Nonviolent Coordinating Committee, the goal of which was to create a "beloved community" while working to end segregation through nonviolence (Ransby, 2003, p. 344).

By the 1970s, although feminists and Civil Rights organizations were working for political rights, medicine, along with other social institutions, was suffering a "stunning loss of confidence" (Starr, 1982, p. 334). Accounts of patient experimentation and unethical treatment challenged the belief that doctors held the patient's best interests in mind. Patient rights became a movement unto itself with particular consumer groups including the aged, African Americans (Black Panthers), gays, and lesbians, as well as women. Sheryl Ruzek notes that in the 1970s, there was already a history of widespread dissatisfaction with conventional obstetric and gynecologic services, "even among the women not actively involved in either the women's health movement or the larger feminist movement" (Ruzek, 1978, p. 9).

Dissatisfaction With Obstetric and Gynecologic Services

In the 1970s, as women became more vocal, they shifted their sights to include gynecologic and reproductive health as a measure of inequity and injustice. The definition of women's health, the question of who should control it, and how to own it became central to the essence of this movement. Harnessing their collective strength in parallel fashion to U.S. civil rights activists, feminists presented an organized challenge to powerful groups, such as the medical profession and hospital administrators (Morgen, 2002).

Women began teaching each other about their bodies and challenging their doctors' decisions in terms of their reproductive and gynecologic health care. Pregnancy and childbirth were considered important feminist life events that did not require unnecessary medical interventions. Rejecting the role of passive patient, women learned to be assertive, ask tough questions, do their own research, insist on certain tests, refuse others, and demand that doctors take their ailments seriously (Morgen, 2002). Thus, women's health grassroots activism became not just a movement but also a discourse.

Women of Color and Reproductive Rights

In a parallel fashion to their interpretation of the overall women's movement, women of color challenged normative definitions of the term *reproductive rights* largely through their ambivalence over abortion rights. As Black activist Angela Davis (1983) contends, White activists frequently overlooked ideological underpinnings of the reproductive rights movement. Before *Roe v. Wade* (1973), most minority women who sought abortion services were forced to do so with backroom abortionists. In fact, several years before the legalization of abortion, New York City witnessed 80% of its deaths from botched abortions as belonging to Black and Puerto Rican women. Davis argues that these women were not so much pro-abortion as they were pro-reproductive rights. In addition, many of the minority women who sought abortions did so because of poor health and living conditions as opposed to their desire to be free of their pregnancy. Through an appreciation of the socially constructed nature of reproductive rights, activists were challenged to gain an important understanding of their various sisters in the cause. This understanding was not always operationalized.

Until the exposure of reproductive rights violations, it was hard for feminists to approach mutual understandings and effective collaborations toward a fully representative reproductive rights platform. Elena R. Gutierrez speaks to this exposure in her challenge to the stereotype of women of Mexican origin as hyper-breeders. By adopting a social constructivist approach to the analysis, Gutierrez turns the cameras around to focus on the institutions that claim ownership of the "problem" of the fertility of Mexican women: demographers, medical professionals, population policy makers, and Chicana feminists (Gutierrez, 2008).

National Women's Health Network

All of these activists challenged how medicine and society viewed the health of women representative of multiple races and classes. By the 1970s, as Berger (2010) argues, social movements experienced both repression as well as periods of experimentation and expansion. The pioneering work of women's groups in the 1960s eventually created a constituency for and shaped the agenda of the National Women's Health Network, formed in 1975 as a national organization dedicated to advancing the health of women of all classes and races through authoritative watchdog organizations, evaluating treatments, research trials, and government policies (Morgen, 2002; Rosen, 2001). At the same time, these same women's health activists, which included nurses, also pushed the controversial borderlands of women's health into public visibility. Issues such as rape, women prisoners, women and mental health, as well as the legalization of prostitution were ideologically challenged in urban cities, such as Philadelphia, for desired reform (Women's Health Concerns Committee [WHCC], Annenberg Rare Book and Manuscript Library).

CASE STUDY: The Maternity Care Coalition—The Philadelpia Story

In the 1980s, the City of Brotherly Love had some of the nation's worst outcomes in terms of infant mortality. Infants in Philadelphia Census Tract 152 were dying at the rate of 34.7 per 1,000, which was almost three times the national rate (12.5%) at the time. An article that appeared in the *Philadelphia Inquirer* on April 5, 1982 was entitled, *5 Blocks that Offer Slimmest Hope to a Baby* (Bishop, 1982). The article shared the grim story of a city where the lack of prenatal care options for marginalized women, in combination with the city's poor coordination and delivery of health services, contributed to the growing phenomenon of poor maternal–child outcomes. It was not until a small group of social justice activists came together to address the issue that the long process to create social change began. The group was known as the MCC and this case study examines the organization's history. The study of family and community health through a historical lens provides powerful insights into problems that continue to exist today. History also allows us to look back and locate and give voice to those people who were on the ground, helping communities develop self-empowerment strategies. Nurses of varying educational level were cornerstones in this history.

(continued)

CASE STUDY: The Maternity Care Coalition—The Philadelpia Story *(continued)*

Leading the Maternity Care Coalition: A Lawyer, a Doctor, and a Nurse Midwife

The totality of energies emerging from the larger women's health movement supplied valuable momentum to Philadelphia's efforts to maximize women's health. Philadelphia's MCC was founded in 1980 and originated as a subcommittee of the Women's Health Concerns Committee. This committee was built with democratic and participatory ideals that sought to include the voices of *all* concerned with women's health. Professionals such as physicians, lawyers, nurses, and policy makers worked with grassroots community members, many of whom were the same women struggling for equitable access to women's health services.

The Southeastern Region of the Pennsylvania Department of Health created the WHCC in the fall of 1974. Its major emphasis rested with the concern that there should be more communication between the government of Pennsylvania and women's organizations (WHCC). Local Philadelphia activists were already discussing the city's high infant mortality rates and how they envisioned meaningful change. The MCC started as a conversation among Edward Sparer, Walter Lear, and Sister Teresita Hinnegan (J. Fisher, oral history interview with L. Maldonado, July 2012). The combination of these three personalities and their professional backgrounds served as a powerful catalyst to the formation of the MCC.

Edward Sparer was a 1959 graduate of Brooklyn Law School and became a pioneer in the fields of poverty and health law. He had an inspiring career as a nationally recognized teacher, scholar, and activist. He was a founder of both the first neighborhood legal services program, Mobilization for Youth Legal Services, in New York City, and the first national support center for legal services work, the Columbia Center on Social Welfare Policy and Law. Sparer was "the intellectual

(continued)

CASE STUDY: The Maternity Care Coalition—The Philadelpia Story *(continued)*

architect of the legal strategy of the welfare rights movement" (Schneider, 2000).

Walter Lear became an activist early in his life. He entered medical school during a time when Jewish and Black applicants were typically turned away, and he soon found himself lobbying for racial equality in the medical profession. During the 1960s, he became inspired by the sit-ins and freedom rides as he continued to work for racial equality in the medical profession. From 1961 to 1963, he was a consultant for the National Urban League, doing research and writing that led to the publication of *Health Care and the Negro Population* in 1965.

Joining Sparer and Lear was Sister Teresita Hinnegan, a Catholic sister and nurse midwife with a master's degree in social work. She also was a University of Pennsylvania nursing instructor and health policy activist and became one of the most influential participants in this grassroots collective. Her life of social justice-related work served as a defining and vital component of her life commitment as a Catholic sister. Sister Teresita's dedication to social movement work is an example of how deep religious identities can serve as pathways to continued participation in a wide range of activist actions. In an oral history interview, Sister Teresita shared some insight into what led her into her life's work of advocating for women. From 1955 to 1969, she worked as a Medical Missions sister with the poor in Bangladesh. She came back to the United States to help her sister who was then alone with two children. It was then that she noticed, "how dysfunctional the system was for women with children to get the help they needed." While helping her sister, Sister Teresita worked as a nurse midwife in a Philadelphia community health center, where she witnessed the lack of health care resources for women living in poverty. These experiences influenced her decision to return to school for a masters in social administration at Temple University. She stated, "I learned a

(continued)

CASE STUDY: The Maternity Care Coalition—The Philadelpia Story *(continued)*

lot, again, about the system and how dysfunctional it was and the change that was needed." Sister Teresita combined her triad of professions—nursing, social work, and ministry—into a forceful tool for understanding and working for social justice (Hinnegan, oral history interview, November 2007).

Sparer, Lear, and Sister Teresita became the intellectual force behind the ideological and tactical beginnings of the MCC in the 1980s. These three activists knew their struggle to reduce infant mortality in Philadelphia had to begin with a purposeful study of the area and the issues. Sister Teresita was given the important foundational role of organizing and conducting the study. Her detailed quantitative and qualitative analyses of Philadelphia's areas of highest infant mortality told the story of a city's failure at effectively providing care for its minority infants (Hinnegan, oral history interview, November 2007).

It also revealed persistent accounts of institutionalized racism as minority women were reportedly turned away from area hospitals if they could not pay a cash deposit before being admitted while in labor to the hospital. The activists, however, often had to use creative methods to expose acts of inequality in some of the area hospitals.

As an example, Sister Teresita and her cohort of fellow activists pretended to be low-income patients calling for obstetrical appointments. In one hospital's case, the admitting clerks asked all the activists for preadmission cash deposits of $1,000. Eventually, with the evidence at hand, the hospital administration conceded this was in fact happening. In many cases, they were turned away due to not having insurance. The MCC activists, under the guidance of Sparer, introduced a lawsuit in 1984 against this hospital. They later settled this lawsuit out of court when the hospital agreed to stop this illegal action (Hinnegan, oral history interview, June 2009).

One of the areas of her study that moved Sister Teresita greatly was the qualitative portion of the study. Sister Teresita

(continued)

CASE STUDY: The Maternity Care Coalition—The Philadelpia Story *(continued)*

and a group of activists surveyed the streets of the two health districts by talking with the women. She said the women had stories to share with the interviewers, stories of how they were treated by hospitals and clinics and how they felt about that treatment. Many of the women shared that, before the survey, no one really took the time to listen to them. One particular woman shared that she "felt like a slab of meat" in the hospital because no one looked upon her as though she was worthy of attention. In a soft voice, Sister Teresita explained why during her oral history—"because nobody cared. Nobody cared." Part of what Sister Teresita and her fellow activists did was to bring these stories of institutionalized racism to city officials. She felt strongly that an important component of MCC's activism was to help these women develop their own voices so they themselves could bring their stories forward, rather than allowing the inequities that weighted them into submission (Hinnegan, oral history interview, June 2009).

Plan for the Provision of Maternity Services in Philadelphia Health Districts 5 and 6

In 1978, Sister Teresita initiated a selective area analysis of Lower North Central Philadelphia (Philadelphia Health Districts 5 and 6) to examine factors that influenced pregnancy outcomes. The study provided a comprehensive look at the two health districts' transportation access, the racial compositions of the neighborhoods, and the number of residential structures that had been vacant for a long period of time, as well as the capital program projects for the areas. She looked at the sites for pregnancy testing and prenatal care, the hospitals used for childbirth in the identified health districts, as well as the low-birth-weight statistics and infant death statistics.

Another important component of the study was a survey of the hospitals from Health Districts 5 and 6 that women used

(continued)

CASE STUDY: The Maternity Care Coalition—The Philadelpia
Story *(continued)*

for their obstetrical services. Sister Teresita asked local neighborhood volunteers to implement one part of the survey. This
component looked at the hospitals in terms of their facilities
and what they offered to patients, such as financial assistance,
educational programs, translation services, and the amount
of sibling and father involvement, as well as rooming in and
breastfeeding support for the women.

Sister Teresita found that women from Health Districts 5
and 6 received inadequate prenatal care and experienced a high
number and rate of low-birth-weight babies as well as a high
rate of infant mortality where the socioeconomic profile of
the area indicated widespread poverty; high unemployment;
underemployment in low-paying dead-end jobs; and low educational achievement. The housing profile indicated that people
were living in environments that had been allowed to dete-
riorate. Attempts to rehabilitate the neighborhoods had been
minimal.

In her study, Sister Teresita acknowledged the influences
of poverty, social deprivation, and low educational levels on
the high incidence of both low-birth-weight babies and high
infant mortality. Quality prenatal care programs were seen
as arbiters; however, many of the low-income women were
not fully accessing and/or using the prenatal services. On the
other hand, the same services lacked the important outreach
programs, support services, and interagency coordination that
linked the pregnant woman with a continuum of care in her
environment.

As a result of the study and the collaborative strength of
MCC, city officials and hospital administrators were pressured into working to resolve the various issues surrounding
Philadelphia's infant mortality. The MCC and Sister Teresita
worked intensively with Philadelphia's communities of mostly
minority and low-income women who were suffering tragi-
cally high rates of infant mortality (Figure 11.1).

(continued)

CASE STUDY: The Maternity Care Coalition—The Philadelpia Story *(continued)*

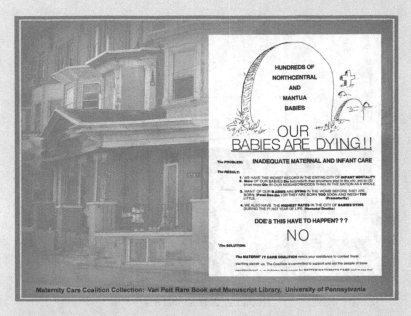

Maternity Care Coalition Collection: Van Pelt Rare Book and Manuscript Library, University of Pennsylvania

FIGURE 11.1 Community action.

Source: Maternity Care Coalition Collection: Van Pelt Rare Book and Manuscript Library, University of Pennsylvania.

MCC, Mom-mobile, and Maternity Care Advocates

The Mom-mobile and the Latina Mom-mobile were MCC's innovative way of reaching into the affected communities within Census Tract 152. Consisting of bright yellow vans staffed by trained community advocates, the Mom-mobile program provided pregnant women with blood pressure checks and assistance in enrolling in prenatal care, Medicaid, food stamps, and other relevant programs. "Maternity Care Advocates" were MCC employees who were also trusted and respected members of the affected communities. In addition to finding pregnant women who were not enrolled in prenatal care, these

(continued)

CASE STUDY: The Maternity Care Coalition—The Philadelpia Story *(continued)*

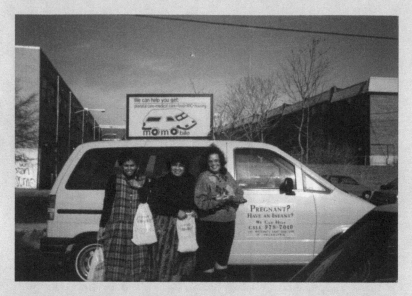

FIGURE 11.2 Mom-mobiles.

Source: Maternity Care Coalition Collection: Van Pelt Rare Book and Manuscript Library, University of Pennsylvania.

advocates also tried to locate and assist homeless and addicted pregnant women (Figure 11.2).

These community advocates were usually older women who resided in the same low-income neighborhoods as well as minority women who had experiential knowledge of the loss of an infant. The notion of using community members toward health promotion is a powerful idea that arose from 1960s groups, such as the Black Panthers and Young Lords. Staffed also with medical assistants, this unique outreach program brought a new kind of health promotion with services, such as pregnancy testing, and subsequent linkage to prenatal care for low-income women in their neighborhoods. In addition to prenatal health promotion, MCC played a crucial role in low-income women's increasing sense of empowerment through

(continued)

CASE STUDY: The Maternity Care Coalition—The Philadelpia Story *(continued)*

various social support programs, such as classes on consumer rights in health care and how to navigate hospital system barriers.

One of the MCC's most effective on the ground activities was its alliance with the Philadelphia Welfare Rights Organization. Dorothy Jordan, a former welfare recipient, became an advocate to the women in the communities MCC served. Jordan rose in the ranks of the welfare rights organization initially by being asked to take over a class on welfare rights in which she was an attendee. In her words, she shared, "my training started on the ground and never looked back" (D. Jordan, oral history interview, December 2012). Eventually, Jordan became involved with the MCC as an advocate. Her role included counseling women who missed prenatal appointments, searching in the communities for women who missed prenatal appointments, recruiting pregnant women into prenatal care, as well as assisting these women to obtain necessary social services, such as food stamps, Women, Infant, and Children (WIC) assistance, and other forms of social support. "There was not just one way to get change" (D. Jordan, oral history interview, December 2012). Maternity care advocates such as Jordan were mature and trusted women from the affected communities who contributed greatly to MCC's vision of bringing the community into awareness of maternal–child health.

Philadelphia's MCC drew its activist representation from both the professional and public realms. Professionals such as nurses, doctors, and social workers attempted to work collaboratively with each other as well as share a mutual commitment to bridging the gap between them and minority communities. A fundamental characteristic of the MCC was a commitment to democratic ideals. This ideal meant the organization was created based on social arrangements that were inclusive of all people regardless of class, race, nationality, ethnicity, gender, or sexual orientation. This also meant a shared understanding

(continued)

CASE STUDY: The Maternity Care Coalition—The Philadelpia Story *(continued)*

that everyone, not just socially recognized experts, was capable of developing constructive ideas. The MCC operationalized the belief that people's ideas are shaped by their location in society, and that those who are located in the marginal positions are particularly capable of thinking insightfully about social problems as well as their own situations. This type of mind-set allowed communities to harness their own sense of power as they assumed ownership of the issues and solutions.

The MCC survived and flourished as a result of strong community engagement and support as well as an inclusive, non-hierarchical, and collaborative style of management. Thirty-two years later, MCC has evolved from an initial staff of three to a staff of more than 100 and from a budget of $116,000 to a budget of $8 million. Looking back, Joanne Fisher, executive director of the MCC, reflects that birth has always attracted her interests, whether it is the birth of an infant or the birth of an organization. Fisher, who got her start with the MCC as a social worker, has seen many challenges and changes within her organization. What continues to challenge Fisher is that she has not seen things get better in terms of the social commitments surrounding childbearing and supporting families (J. Fisher, oral history interview, July 2012).

DISCUSSION AND CONCLUSION

The MCC considered the cause of high infant mortality rates in Philadelphia as arising from a combination of factors. Hospital systems' failures coupled with marginalized communities' lack of education, resources, and social support were viewed as foundational to the problem. As advocates surveyed women on the streets of Philadelphia and listened to their stories, they quickly learned of the institutionalized forms of racism occurring in the city. Issues of heath disparities were recognized as issues of social equity. Many low-income, marginalized women received prejudicial treatment in medical institutions that in turn prompted the activists to confront these institutions directly. At times, the negotiations became contentious. The activists employed a grassroots style of participatory democracy in which all members of society as well as the affected communities were invited to join the activism to change the landscape these women faced.

Over time, Philadelphia infant mortality rates slowly declined. For example, in 1990, Health District 5 infant mortality rate was 21.2 per 1,000 live births (Copeland, 1992). Major accomplishments of the MCC were its strong advocacy and social support to communities of marginalized women. The trust the organization garnered from the affected communities fostered the women's self-empowerment process. Women felt they owned and held control over their health as opposed to it belonging to uncaring health systems. They learned to negotiate with health care systems as well as learned their rights as health care consumers. Once the momentum of education, support, and advocacy was started, community members became leaders in the process. The results were changes in both macro and micro systems surrounding the women. Ultimately, with this high touch, highly collaborative style of organizing, the women in the communities became self-empowered to seek and expect quality prenatal care.

The study of family and community health through a historical lens can provide powerful insights into present-day problems that are reflected not only in health care systems but also in our nursing education programs. In terms of our health care system, history allows us to look back to consider how a community's sociopolitical context affected health. Ultimately, we can develop strategies for the present based on our lessons from the past. Community engagement and nursing, once considered a radical idea, is now being taught as well as instituted (Israel, Schulz, Parker, & Becker, 2011).

Currently, engaging with communities is not only an emerging theme within health and social policy circles, but also within nursing academic programs. For example, the University of Pennsylvania School of Nursing conducts its clinical experiences within West Philadelphia. This city neighborhood is where the students live, practice, and currently engage with their neighbors in partnerships that encourage healthier outcomes (D'Antonio, Walsh Brennan, & Curley, 2013). Lessons from the past clearly outline the knowledge, skills, and attitudes necessary to assume successful community leadership roles.

ACTIVITIES FOR TEACHING AND LEARNING

1. Discuss infant mortality as a relevant contemporary issue and relate it to the history of social justice and women's health.
2. Discuss the political legacy of women's health and the struggle women have endured to own and control their health themselves.

REFERENCES

About.com. (2016). Women's history. Retrieved from http://womenshistory .about.com/od/laws/a/comstock_law.htm

Berger, D. (2010). *The hidden 1970s: Histories of radicalism*. New Brunswick, NJ: Rutgers University Press.

Bishop, M. (1982, April 5). 5 blocks that offer slimmest hope to a baby. *Philadelphia Inquirer*, 1–8.

Burwell v. Hobby Lobby Stores, 573 U.S. ___ (2014).

Copeland, L. (1992). Study tries to explain baby death rates they vary by neighborhood in the city: The Health Department Report cites obstacles to prenatal care. Retrieved from http://articles.philly.com/1992-07-15/news/ 26026627_1_infant-mortality-infant-death-prenatal-care

D'Antonio, P., Walsh Brennan, A. M., & Curley, M. (2013). Judgment, inquiry, engagement, voice: Reenvisioning an undergraduate nursing curriculum using a shared decision-making model. *Journal of Professional Nursing, 29*(6), 407–413.

Griswold v. Connecticut, 381 U.S. 479 (1965).

Gutierrez, E. R. (2008). *Fertile matters: The politics of Mexican-origin women's reproduction*. Austin, TX: University of Texas Press.

Harrington, M. (1962). *The other America: Poverty in the United States*. New York, NY: Simon & Schuster.

Hewitt, N. A. (Ed.). (2010). *No permanent waves: Recasting histories of U.S. feminism*. New Brunswick, NJ: Rutgers University Press.

Hinnegan, Sister Teresita. *Plan for the provision of maternity services in Health Districts 5 and 6 (Lower North Central Philadelphia)*. Personal papers, 4–6.

Israel, B. A., Schulz, A. J., Parker, E. A., & Becker, A. B. (2011). Community-based participatory research: Policy recommendations for promoting a partnership approach in health research. *Education for Health, 14*(2), 182–197.

Lear, W. (2007). U.S. health professionals oppose war. *Social Medicine, 2*(3), 131–135.

Lewenson, S. (1993). *Taking charge: Nursing, suffrage, and feminism 1873–1920.* New York, NY: Garland Publishing.

Lynaugh, J. (1991). The death of Sadie Sachs. *Nursing Research, 40*(2), 124–125.

Morgen, S. (2002). *Into our own hands: The women's health movement in the United States.* New Brunswick, NJ: Rutgers University Press.

Ransby, B. (2003). *Ella Baker & The Black Freedom Movement: A radical democratic vision.* Chapel Hill: University of North Carolina Press.

Roe v. Wade, 410 U. S. 113 (1973).

Rosen, R. (2001). *The world split open: How the modern women's movement changed America.* New York, NY: Penguin Group.

Ruzek, S. (1978). *The women's health movement.* New York, NY: Praeger.

Sanger, M. (1938). *An Autobiography.* New York, NY: W. W. Norton.

Schneider, E. M. (2000). Fifteenth anniversary of the Edward V. Sparer Public Interest Law Fellowship Program. (2000). *Brooklyn Law Review, 66,* 147–151.

Schoen, J. (2005). *Choice and coercion: Birth control, sterilization, and abortion in public health and welfare.* Chapel Hill: University of North Carolina Press.

Springer, K. (2005). *Living for the revolution: Black feminist organizations, 1968–1980.* Durham, NC: Duke University Press.

Women's Health Concerns Committee. (1980). Women's Health Collection (MS 588. Box 20, Folder 284). Annenberg Rare Book & Manuscript Library, University of Pennsylvania, PA.

Index

Printed in the United States
By Bookmasters